- **Are my headaches caused by tension—or something else?**

- **Should I be concerned about my chest pains?**

- **Are my monthly mood swings *really* "all in my head"?**

- **Why do I have so much trouble sleeping?**

Some ailments—even common ones—are especially difficult to recognize. A wide array of puzzling and confusing symptoms can lead doctors to misdiagnose a patient's problem—and prescribe inappropriate and ineffective treatment. This book describes many such ailments and offers easy-to-understand explanations to help you relieve your symptoms. If you've been to doctor after doctor and still haven't found a satisfactory answer—this is the book for you...

**SYMPTOMS & SOLUTIONS**

*How to Tell When
Your Ailments Are Misdiagnosed—
and What to Do About It*

# SYMPTOMS &SOLUTIONS

## JAY A. GOLDSTEIN, M.D.

Published in hardcover as *Could Your Doctor Be Wrong?*

BERKLEY BOOKS, NEW YORK

Published in hardcover as *Could Your Doctor Be Wrong?*

## IMPORTANT NOTE

Medicine is an ever-changing science. As new research and clinical experience broaden
our knowledge, changes in treatment and drug therapy are required. Although many suggestions for drug usages are made in it, this book is intended for educational purposes
only, and the author, editor, and publisher do not accept liability in the event of negative
consequences incurred as a result of information presented herein. We do not claim that
this information is necessarily accurate by the rigid, scientific standard applied for medical proof and therefore make no warranty, express or implied, with respect to the material herein contained. Therefore the patient is urged to consult his or her own physician
prior to following a course of treatment. The reader must bear in mind that this book is
not for the purposes of self-diagnosis or self-treatment and that any and all medical problems should be referred to the expertise of appropriate medical personnel.

Physicians are urged to check the product information sheet included in the pack-
age of each drug they plan to administer to be certain the protocol followed is not
in conflict with the manufacturer's inserts. When a discrepancy arises between these
inserts and information in this book, the physician is encouraged to use his or her
best professional judgment.

This Berkley book contains the complete text of the original hardcover edition. It
has been completely reset in a typeface designed for easy reading and was printed
from new film.

### SYMPTOMS & SOLUTIONS

A Berkley Book / published by arrangement with
Pharos Books

PRINTING HISTORY
Pharos Books edition published 1991
Berkley edition / February 1993

ISBN: 0-425-13627-2

A BERKLEY BOOK ® ™ 757,375
Berkley Books are published by The Berkley Publishing Group,
200 Madison Avenue, New York, New York 10016.
The name "BERKLEY" and the "B" logo
are trademarks belonging to Berkley Publishing Corporation.

PRINTED IN THE UNITED STATES OF AMERICA

10 9 8 7 6 5 4 3 2

**To Gail,
without whose help
and inspiration
I would never have
written this book.**

# Contents

# Introduction

I am a doctor of last resort. In my practice over the last few years I have seen thousands of patients with a wide diversity of illnesses, many of whom had almost given up hope.

Typically, before getting to me, they have seen four or five—sometimes as many as a dozen—different doctors, all without receiving relief. Their most common complaint is "My other doctors tell me it's 'all in my head.' They just don't help me."

Is this possible? In an age when medicine has advanced further in diagnosing disorders in the last fifty years than in the previous five thousand, is it really possible that all these people are imagining their illnesses?

I think not.

While there are doctors who look for innovative solutions to the problems their patients have, I believe that there is also a large group of physicians who prefer to follow the medical "cookbook" they received as part of their training.

This medical cookbook, as I call it, is at the core of the problem. It lists all commonly known diseases with their symptoms and treatments. It tells the physician, for example, how to diagnose appendicitis and what to do for the patient who has this illness.

The problem, however, is that a great many disorders are not included. For example, premenstrual syndrome (PMS) was not part of the cookbook until perhaps ten years ago. Prior to that, women with this problem were told they were imagining their symptoms. Even today some doctors still don't believe that PMS exists, and PMS is only slowly finding its way into the medical cookbook. There are many disorders like PMS that have only gained partial acceptance.

And a great many illnesses are not even included at all in most doctors' cookbook. For example, if you go to your doctor with a headache, he may well know what to do if it's caused by a brain lesion or a classic migraine. But a minority of headaches are caused by these disorders. The rest may receive a prescription for pain pills and the patient is told to "live with it" or "perhaps you have too much stress."

Or what if you have Chronic Fatigue Syndrome (CFS), a disease that is almost at epidemic proportions in this country? Until 1988 the vast majority of doctors refused to even acknowledge its existence. Only when the Centers for Disease Control in Atlanta confirmed its existence and came up with a working definition of the illness did some physicians begin to believe it really exists. Even today, if you go to your doctor with symptoms of CFS, the chances are you'll be told you're suffering from depression and perhaps be referred to a psychiatrist.

Unless your problem has clear medical-cookbook symptoms and responds to medical-cookbook treatment, many (perhaps most) physicians don't really want to deal with it—or with you. If it's not in the cookbook, most doctors seem to say it doesn't exist. Somehow, most physicians never seem to think that the cookbook itself could be inadequate.

But many illnesses don't fit the cookbook model. And most people at one time or another have one of these problems, among them:

Undefined abdominal pain
Asthma
Chronic fatigue
Chest pain not associated with heart trouble
Depression
Headache
Impotence
Lower back pain
PMS (premenstrual syndrome)
Chronic sinusitis
Sleep disorders
Chronic sore throat

These conditions often present confusing and puzzling symptoms. The cookbook physician may try to sift through and make them fit a diagnosis with which he or she is comfortable, then prescribe a series of tests to confirm the diagnosis.

Of course, if the original diagnosis was incorrect, the tests will not confirm it. I cannot begin to count the number of times patients tell me that their tests are all normal. Of course they are normal; they were the wrong tests (or there may be no objective test to make the diagnosis)!

When the tests don't reveal anything and the cookbook doesn't give any more help, many physicians become extremely uncomfortable. You as a patient are presenting a challenge. Rather than believing you and trying to figure out for themselves what might truly be wrong, too often they'd rather refer you to someone else. Referrals are much easier than trying to figure out what the problem is.

The trouble with this, however, is that you get bounced around, often at great expense and sometimes at great pain. And too often, you don't get real help.

This is not to condemn all physicians or medicine in general. It is to say, however, that there are problems with medicine today. There are large holes in the practice of medicine as it is carried out in this country. When you go to your doctor, if he is not an enlightened and creative healer or if you don't have a cookbook illness, you may not get the best treatment.

In defense of most physicians, the amount of knowledge needed to practice general medicine has expanded so rapidly that many believe it is now impossible for one person to know enough to do an adequate job. Furthermore, the threat of malpractice suits and possible insurance nonreimbursement deters the physician from dealing with patients who have difficult problems.

## WHAT WENT WRONG

How could this situation have come about? The common wisdom is that the physician is the healer, who has gone through years and years of training. How is it possible that this person might not have all the answers, especially answers that are available elsewhere?

The best way to answer this question is to tell you a story. In 1964, when I entered medical school, physicians were highly respected and were generally regarded as always putting the interests of the patient ahead of their own. It was fairly difficult to gain admission to American medical schools, which tended to attract the "best and the brightest" of college students. Malpractice suits were uncommon and, at least in the naive viewpoint of my classmates and myself, one practiced medicine to help people and to be intellectually stimulated. (I cannot think of a single member of my class who chose a specialty based on the amount of money to be made.)

In addition, after World War II a scientific revolution had occurred in medicine, and research and teaching became a national priority. It was assumed that the physician knew best, and in those days I rarely heard of any medical insurance claim being denied, no matter how preposterous it may have seemed. Medicare and Medicaid, fairly new programs then, were working well and compensated physicians adequately.

Most of us viewed becoming a doctor much like entering the priesthood. We had the sacred obligation to learn as much as possible to help the patient to the utmost of our ability—without, of course, betraying society's trust to act in an ethical and professional manner at all times.

That era, which lasted into the mid-1970s, is now regarded as the Golden Age of medicine by those of us old enough to remember it. Unfortunately, it had a great flaw that was not apparent at the time. That flaw was that there was no specialty of "generalization."

GPs (general practitioners) were considered mentally deficient bumpkins. No one in my graduating glass went into general practice. There wasn't even an area of family medicine, as there is today.

In other words, medicine became specialized, one might even say "organ-specific." There were doctors to take care of your gall bladder and your heart and your kidneys. But no doctors to take care of nonspecific abdominal pain or chronic fatigue.

As medicine became more specialized, there was less and less integration of knowledge among the various specialists. Today, since the general knowledge base of medicine has grown so dramatically, this problem has reached acute proportions.

## PSYCHIATRY—THE MOST CRITICAL DEFICIENCY

Looking back now, I believe that the most critical deficiency of that era of fragmentation was in psychiatry. Psychiatry was the ideal discipline to offer the hope of a whole-body, integrated approach to medicine.

Unfortunately, at the time psychiatry was completely dominated by psychoanalysts. Psychoanalysis had become included in medicine and had gained a degree of respectability, even though the discipline remained generally incomprehensible to the majority of physicians.

The truth is that psychoanalysis has few scientific or experimental underpinnings and is so complicated and arcane a study that many psychiatrists trying to absorb this mass of esoterica knew little about other forms of psychotherapy. Few understood the physiology of the brain or the emerging disciplines of behavior modification or of biological psychiatry.

As a result, the promise psychiatry offered of being a discipline that would *integrate* all of the body in a unified approach to medicine was not fulfilled.

## A CASE HISTORY

Here is an example of what I mean. It involved a new approach to treating delusions that I developed early in my career. (Eventually I published a description of this technique in a professional journal, but the initial reaction from my peers was far from positive.)

This approach, new at the time, involved *convincing* patients to give up their delusions. (A delusion is a false belief—in this case, that you are someone else, a famous person, and possess that person's power.) My first case was my most memorable one. I was called to the psychiatric emergency area by an admitting resident who knew I wanted to treat a patient with a delusion in a new way. The police had brought in a patient who had been hospitalized before with the delusion that he was Julius Caesar. He was dressed in toga, sandals, and a laurel wreath. The ward staff knew what I wanted them to do, and the ward chief psychiatrist had a convenient laissez-faire attitude toward my inventions.

When the patient was ushered into my office I was wrapped in a sheet, toga fashion, and I exclaimed, "Hail Caesar! I'm Brutus."

"Brutus? I thought you were Dr. Goldstein!" he replied.

"That's what they think," I said conspiratorially.

"When do we take over the world?" he asked.

"I'm waiting for the message from the flying saucer," I replied, feeling it was important to play along, but also to one-up him each time I was challenged.

After a short time he began to believe me. I then pointed out that the only difference between our current situations was that I wasn't going to tell anyone that I was Brutus until the right time. Until then, people thought I was Dr. Goldstein. I made a good living, had friends, and was respected in the community. I contrasted my situation to his: He had no money, no friends, he had been arrested for vagrancy and was now landing in the looney bin. The only difference was that he told people who he "really" was and I didn't. I suggested that he pretend he was Richard Roe (not his real name) until we heard from the flying saucer, and that we make up some kind of story about why he thought he was Julius Caesar.

"I could tell them I took some LSD," he said, getting into the spirit of the deception. The ward staff knew that they should reinforce his new identity of Richard Roe by being friendly to him, laughing at his jokes, and so on. This inter-action occurred on a Friday afternoon and I went home for the weekend.

First thing Monday morning we had ward rounds, where we visited all the patients and discussed each case. We would then tell the ward chief what was happening with our patients. But that morning the regular ward chief wasn't there; the assistant superintendent of the hospital had taken his place.

Still, I did not foresee any problem with my treatment of Richard Roe, because I couldn't see how any therapy could have made him any worse. What I had done, although it may sound like improvisational theater, was actually based on an ingenious type of treatment called cognitive disso-nance therapy, in which the therapist attempts to make the patient's beliefs seem not in his best interests, something like the cognitive therapy of Aaron Beck, which is popular and effective today.

To my surprise, the assistant superintendent became very upset and asked that the patient, whom I had not seen or spoken to since Friday, be brought into the meeting room. Richard came in, behavior and dress quite appropriate. "I hear you're Julius Caesar," the psychiatrist said. "That's what I used to think before I met Dr. Goldstein," Richard said, as I heaved a sigh of relief. For the next hour the psychiatrist tried to convince Richard that he really was Julius Caesar, but he wouldn't budge. Then he had Richard leave. And for the next ninety minutes the assistant superintendent excoriated me for deviating from the orthodox treatment. (The orthodox cookbook treatment, by the way, had never worked.)

Richard left the hospital in a few days, and right before he did he thanked me. "I realize now what you were doing, Dr. Goldstein," he said. "But I like being Richard Roe better than Julius Caesar, and I'll try to make my life work this way." We never saw him at the hospital again.

If there is a moral to this story, it's that some changes come very slowly in medicine, perhaps too slowly. I was chastised not for hurting a patient—indeed, I had helped him—but for doing something new. No credit was given to the fact that it worked. Perhaps this story will begin to bring home the problems with medicine that I am discussing.

There is a great emphasis today on using diagnostic and therapeutic methods that have been proved effective by numerous experiments. Many physicians and insurance companies believe that any approach which does not meet these standards should not be used. It is difficult for me to agree with this viewpoint except to say that, in an era of decreasing funds available for medical research, appropriate experiments for every rational new idea are difficult if not impossible to perform.

Furthermore, since we have limited resources to meet the health-care needs of the nation, a problem that has only become critical in the last decade, some middle ground must be found between doing everything a physician thinks might ideally benefit his patient and having the resources available to do it.

For this reason, one of the growth industries in medicine recently has been "outcome research" to assess what might be the most cost-effective ways of managing various problems.

This sort of research is good in that it sets a uniform standard for medical practice but bad in that deviation from this standard is discouraged, if not condemned.

## CHANGES COMING

Fortunately, change is beginning to happen. For example, psychiatry now acknowledges that the brain is indeed connected to the body. This permits the use of all sorts of new and helpful techniques, such as behavioral and biological therapy. Unfortunately, many medical specialists, even those who now accept this fact, have little idea how the brain itself works. As more and more evidence accumulates, ignoring the discoveries in the mind–body relationship will become increasingly difficult.

## MONEY AND DOCTORS

Then there is the matter of money. Over a decade or more the economics of medicine has changed dramatically, due in part to the emergence of corporate medicine and of the "me generation" of doctors.

Today, unlike when I was a medical student, the top medical-school graduates tend not to go into research but into areas where the economic rewards are greater. Yet they are the ones most ideally suited to treat "difficult" patients, those with illnesses which do not fit the cookbook; they should be the family practitioners and general internists. They have the all-round general knowledge and the curiosity to make an unusual diagnosis and come up with a novel but effective treatment.

Unfortunately, there is little economic incentive in the current medical system for the best students to go into general medicine. The remuneration is low, compared to procedure-oriented specialties. Changes are beginning to be made to redress the inequity, but it will probably always remain. Medical students are also deterred from a career in general medicine because it is considered too broad and the responsibilities to patients too time-consuming. Young physicians seem to be more aware that there is life outside medical practice than my contemporaries were.

## THE WEAKNESS OF AMERICAN PHYSICIANS

To adequately deal with the *whole* body one must truly become a superior physician. This requires mastery of general medicine as well as substantial knowledge of a wide variety of specialized areas such as virology, immunology, biological psychiatry, pharmacology, molecular biology, and pain management. Unfortunately, most of these areas are those in which American physicians are notoriously weak.

To have an adequate understanding of these disciplines requires many more years of study than most physicians are willing or able to commit to. The sad truth is that most doctors today want to finish school, internship, and residency as quickly as possible so that they can get out there and start earning "doctor's pay."

**NOT WANTING TO TAKE THE TIME TO LEARN** For several years I taught family practice residents at several well-known medical centers in Southern California. Many of the residents I met were highly intelligent and dedicated, but an alarming number saw their training as getting a ticket punched to board certification.

In my own training, I was accustomed to working with young doctors who wanted to learn all they could and who would redouble their efforts if they did not know enough about a certain disease they encountered on rounds. As a teacher, however, I was totally unprepared for the attitude of some young doctors who did not care if a gap in understanding occurred. I was disappointed and even horrified by those who did not even want to learn how to think like a doctor. I believed that some of these residents were so morally and intellectually unfit to be physicians that I actually feared for the safety of their patients!

Increasingly money, the bottom line, is the thing that matters most to doctors. For a long time, physicians were given the responsibility to put the needs of the patients ahead of their own finances. It was thought that doctors would not try to realize monetary gain by ordering tests or doing procedures that were not warranted. But this attitude mattered less and less as time progressed. Medicine became increasingly a business. During this period reimbursement to physicians from insurance companies declined as costs skyrocketed, putting more pressure on the practitioner to be aware of the dollars involved in what he was doing. It has become more difficult for the unscrupulous physician to exploit the system, but at the same time more difficult for the idealistic physician to be innovative.

## WHAT THIS MEANS TO YOU

What this means is that when you present your doctor with symptoms that are in any way out of the ordinary, you may get an incorrect diagnosis. If your problem fits the cookbook, then your diagnosis and treatment will probably be appropriate and effective.

But beyond the scope of the medical cookbook is a vast gray area. Your physician may insist on your having a large number of tests and X-rays. When these tests come out "normal" (because, as I noted earlier, they may have been the wrong tests) your doctor may shake his head at your continued complaints and suggest, "It's all in your head!" Other doctors you are referred to, also going by the cookbook, may come to the same conclusion. In the end, you may begin to doubt your own sanity.

## FINDING THE RIGHT DOCTOR

This does not mean, however, that there are no doctors out there who can and will treat your illness effectively. There are, but many people are unable to distinguish between a cookbook doctor and one who is innovative and dedicated to healing.

How do you find the right doctor? Here are some clues:

*First,* look for the generalist. A specialist can be a good generalist, but more likely this person is a general internist or family physician. The important point is that he or she accepts a wide variety of patients and complaints, not just a small, narrow, specialized group.

Ask to see your doctor's credentials; discuss them. Ask about your doctor's approach to medicine, why he or she became a doctor. An enlightened generalist will discuss with you the ideas he is testing.

*Second,* you want to have a doctor you can talk to. The

doctor's financial and time constraints keep the amount of time available to you at a minimum. However, during that time you should be able to discuss alternative diagnoses and treatments. The doctor should acknowledge that there's no one more interested in your illness and its cure than you. He or she should be willing to spend the time to explain why a particular course of action might or might not be fruitful.

Speak at length with your doctor about your problem. You should not tolerate a physician who is too busy to hear what you have to say. If a course of treatment is not working, ask your doctor if he has considered other possibilities. (But remember that your physician must also practice cost-effective medicine, and you will be charged for the time he spends with you.)

Beware of the doctor who dismisses everything out of hand and who doesn't want to get into the unusual symptoms you may have. Your "unusual symptoms" may actually be the clues to solving your problem. And beware of any doctor who says, in whatever terms, "It's all in your head!"

*Third,* your doctor should come up with ideas without prompting. If what he's doing isn't making you better, he should be trying different things. By this, I don't mean that he keep sending you out for test after test, but rather that he explain to you the approach he's taking. This is only logical.

*Fourth,* carefully consider your priorities. It is important to like your doctor and also helpful if he is conveniently located. But some of the best doctors may be irascible. They may be hard to get along with, but perhaps they can help you. They may also have so many patients that you'll have to wait a week or two to get in. But the wait may be worthwhile if you get well.

Look for a physician who will listen carefully and be able to apply a broad base of knowledge to your problem to come up with a sound diagnosis and appropriate treatment.

Above all, don't settle for second-best medicine. If you have a problem, you deserve to have it considered for what it is. If your doctor tries to make your problem fit a cookbook diagnosis, he's doing you a disservice.

## COULD YOUR DOCTOR BE WRONG?

Given the state of medicine today, if you find that your doctor begins to treat you as though you are cranky, a pest, or a complainer, do not assume that the problem is necessarily with you. Your complaints could be you acting in your own best interests. You are only trying to communicate that you are not well and your doctor's reaction may be caused by his frustration because he cannot help you.

Of course, this is not to suggest that you should establish an adversarial relationship with your doctor. That's not going to help you get better. What you need to do, instead, is to recognize some of the limitations of modern medicine and modern physicians. Then you should plan a course of action that will result in your getting better.

One avenue to pursue is to go through this book and find the areas that may touch on your problem. I have indicated alternative diagnoses as well as numerous alternative treatments.

Many of these remedies are not of the self-help kind. To apply them you need a doctor who will work with you. Show the doctor this book and discuss the therapies and diagnoses it mentions. This book contains treatments that many physicians won't have considered.

My goal in this book is to give you, the patient, both a clearer understanding of your medical problem and what should be appropriate treatment. Then you can compare this approach with what your doctor has said and done. You should then be able to judge whether or not your doctor might be wrong, and you can discuss your concerns with him or her.

Do not expect any doctor to be perfect. All of us make mistakes; all of us have our failings. But if you have an innovative physician who is willing to work with you, together you may find the road to good health.

# 1
## Dealing With Pain

We all experience pain on occasion. But, especially for those who live with it day and night, it is not a friendly companion.

When most of us get pain, we seek immediate relief. This is usually accomplished by removing the cause of the pain. Remove the splinter in your finger and, after a short time, the pain will go away.

But for some there is no simple remedy. Chronic back pain or cancer pain, for example, can take on a life of its own. Chronic pain, although obviously a symptom, can become a disorder in itself.

For those suffering chronic unrelieved pain, "It is the best of times, it is the worst of times" these days. More can be done than ever before to relieve your pain. Yet too few patients receive adequate treatment.

### REASONS FOR INADEQUATE PAIN TREATMENT

First, it may be difficult for you to find pain medicine specialists. Relatively few doctors are trained in this new specialty.

Second, treatment can be expensive. Insurance companies are not inclined to pay for pain treatment unrelated to a specific "cookbook" disorder. As a result, few people are likely to seek out those pain clinics that might bring relief but that also might cost much of their personal funds.

Third, many physicians have had little or no training in dealing with chronic pain. Their remedies may be appropriate to short-term solutions such as prescribing a pain-relieving drug, which if addictive can produce more harm than good in the long run.

Finally, the patient him- or herself may be part of the problem. For example, if you have lower back pain and go to a physician, you may expect to be given some pain pills or muscle relaxants and believe the problem will go away in a few days. But the problem may last for months or even years, and pain pills are not the answer in this situation. Yet many people expect immediate relief in the form of miracle pills. Thus we unwittingly put pressure on doctors to give us what we want, even though it may not be the proper treatment. Unfortunately too, some doctors succumb to their patients' demands. Others do not want to deal with chronic pain at all, since it is difficult for some doctors to care for patients who do not get better.

If you suffer from chronic pain, you may feel unsupported and not believed, that your doctor isn't really helping. You may very well be right.

## GETTING HELP

What can you do when you have chronic severe pain?

First, let's talk about the pain itself. Pain is usually a symptom of some underlying problem. In the case of a cookbook illness, most physicians can treat the disorder and thereby relieve the pain.

But what should you do if your physician doesn't seem able to help? He or she may not arrive at a diagnosis that makes sense, at least to you, or a plan of treatment that works. Instead your physician may say "You'll just have to live with pain. Here are some pills that will help keep it down." But the pills may not really help because the basic problem is not being addressed. What are you to do now?

I suggest that you take two courses of action. The most immediate, of course, is to finish reading this chapter, which will give you some understanding of modern pain-treatment techniques. The second is to search out a pain specialist. In larger communities these physicians are often associated with hospitals and may run pain-management clinics. In smaller communities, you may need to investigate whether there is a doctor who has a particular interest in pain management. Ask other doctors for recommendations or call a local physicians' referral board.

## UNDERSTANDING PAIN

There are numerous types of pain and their causes and remedies vary. The simplest is when an area of your body hurts because of injury or from inflammation, possibly due to infection. When a part of the body is traumatized, pain-transmitting nerves are stimulated and send messages to the brain. The result is that you experience pain.

Treating the injury, inflammation, or infection will usually stop the stimulation of the pain-transmitting nerves and the pain will be removed.

However, sometimes it is not directly possible to treat the cause of pain. Back pain or pain from an internal organ such as the pancreas are situations where immediate relief may not be available.

**BREAKING THE PAIN PATH**   When the cause cannot be readily eliminated, an attempt can be made to block transmission of pain signals by the nerves. In the case of a bad cut, an anesthetic may be injected right into the wound, thus temporarily relieving the pain and allowing the physician to clean and suture it.

Another technique is to block the nerves that carry the pain from the site to the spinal cord and the brain by injecting a local anesthetic into the nerve. Although this may seem like a very temporary solution, sometimes it has a lasting benefit. When these procedures are done repeatedly, a feedback cycle (in which the cause of the pain sends signals to the brain, which then produces a bodily reaction such as stiffening, which may cause even more pain) may be interrupted. Thus the injections may actually produce long-term relief of the pain.

Another technique for blocking the transmission of pain is transcutaneous electrical nerve stimulation (TENS). TENS uses a small device that electrically stimulates larger nerves that go into the spinal cord to block out the impulses transmitted through smaller nerves. Battery electrodes are placed at appropriate locations on the patient's body and then repetitive minor shocks occur. Only a mild sensation is felt (although too much current can produce involuntary muscle jerking) and the pain often decreases. The benefit may last for some hours after the treatment has ended. TENS may be used for long periods of time.

Acupuncture is another method that may block the transmission of pain. In acupuncture needles are inserted at specific points in the body to block pain transmission. If the thought of having needles stuck into your body bothers you, you should be aware of the fact that several acupuncture techniques do not involve needle insertion, among them laser stimulation of the acupuncture points, electrical stimulation, or *acupressure.*

There are also methods of directly altering the transmission of pain into the spinal cord. These include surgical approaches that interrupt nerve roots to the part of the spinal cord that is thought to transmit the pain. These more radical approaches should only be considered as a last resort.

Finally, there is a considerable amount of interest in the chemicals that either help or hinder the transmission of pain at the area of the spinal cord in which the nerves enter (the *dorsal horn*). Altering the balance of these chemicals in this region actually determines to what extent pain signals will be received and reacted to by the spinal cord and the brain.

We know about many different chemicals involved in pain transmission in the brain and spinal cord and we are learning about new ones all the time. We also have many drugs that affect these chemicals and may reduce pain, including antidepressants, opioids (opium- or morphinelike drugs), and anticonvulsants.

These methods of dealing with pain are available to all physicians, but not all physicians are equally aware of them or are prepared to use them. You may need to find a specialist in pain who will work with you in determining which is most appropriate for your problem. Unfortunately, chronic pain is an undertreated area of medicine.

## PAIN SYNDROMES

In addition to simple pain, for which there is a readily identifiable (though not necessarily treatable) cause, there are also a variety of pain syndromes which may cause physicians much difficulty in diagnosing. For example, you have a pain in your head and you go to your physician, who examines you but can find no detectable injury or inflammation. Your physician looks puzzled for a moment, then prescribes some pain pills. They help—momentarily. But your problem doesn't go away. What do you do now?

If you don't have an obvious cause for pain that can be treated easily, you may have a *pain syndrome*. Your doctor may continue trying to treat the locale of the pain even though the cause may not be at that site.

The two pain syndromes we talk about here are *fibromyalgia* and *myofascial pain syndrome*. Each requires a different kind of treatment, and you may have to seek out a pain specialist to get that treatment.

**TENDER POINTS** Fibromyalgia, one of the most common of the pain syndromes, is a disorder a great many people experience. It has recently been defined as involving, for diagnostic purposes, eighteen tender points in widely spread locations on both sides of the body. You may feel pain on the left and right sides and in the lower and upper half of the body.

These tender points are not strained or "knotted" muscles that result from overexertion. They are not old tears in cartilage or other underlying structures. If this were the case, in a short time, when the muscles heal, the pain would be gone or would localize.

**TREATING FIBROMYALGIA PAIN** Tender points are usually treated with drugs, but your doctor is limited by standard medical practice in treating your fibromyalgia.* Hence, if your doctor takes the standard approach, the treatments will probably be limited to tricyclic antidepressants, a relative of which is called cyclobenzaprine (Flexeril) and a combination of alprazolam (Xanax) and ibuprofen (Motrin, Advil, etc.). Beyond that, he can offer you little help besides physical therapy and suggesting that you gradually start to exercise. None of these treatments may help you very much, although they may be quite effective for certain patients.

*Standard practice means a treatment that has been proved by double-blind experiments. While these double-blind experiments, in which one set of subjects is given the drug and another a placebo, do truly establish effectiveness, there is simply not enough time or enough money to perform them for all applications of every drug.

On the other hand, I am going to suggest one therapy that you will want to talk over with your physician. While the medications are not proven remedies for fibromyalgia, they may offer you some relief.

**SEROTONIN**   Serotonin is a nerve transmitter (a chemical that helps nerves transmit their messages) thought to be involved in fibromyalgia. Levels of this substance may be low if you have the disorder and raising them may help reduce symptoms. The antidepressant fluoxetine (Prozac) has a very specific serotonin-raising property and is sometimes helpful in treating fibromyalgia. Your doctor should begin it at a low dosage, since you could be sensitive to it. Another medication that affects serotonin is buspirone (Buspar), generally used to treat anxiety. Buspar may be given alone or in combination with Prozac.

## MYOFASCIAL PAIN SYNDROME

An illness related to fibromyalgia and often confused with it is myofascial pain syndrome. In myofascial pain syndrome the tender points are triggers that shoot pain off to some other area of the body—the causes of referred pain.* (The difference between the two is somewhat muddled by the fact that myofascial pain syndrome can "spread" and become fibromyalgia.)

Both conditions are related to tender points or tender nodules in muscles. Tender points cause localized pain. Trigger points (TrPs) cause referred pain.

Unfortunately, the complexity of myofascial pain syndrome is not as well recognized as it should be. Many doctors only concentrate on the site of the pain and do not look for TrPs. These physicians, faced with a mysterious pain problem, may give you injections of a local anesthetic and a cortisone-containing drug directly into the tender areas where muscles attach to bone or into the joint itself. This is particularly true for the shoulder (bursitis) or elbow (tennis elbow).

Sometimes these injections give relief, sometimes they

*Referred (or "transferred") pain is felt in areas at a distance from the site of origin. The pain may follow a spinal nerve or may be felt in a manner that is difficult to understand anatomically.

do not. (Cortisone injections into joints are common in the treatment of certain kinds of arthritis but must be used sparingly.)

I have found the muscles along the lower spine to most frequently be the cause of the abdominal pain involved with myofascial pain syndrome, the superficial more than the deep. Frequently, I have eliminated supposed "gallbladder" or "appendicitis" pain by injecting the appropriate TrPs.

## UNDERSTANDING TRIGGER POINTS

During the last few years a relatively small number of rheumatologists and specialists in physical medicine have been working on the problem of referred pain and have come a long way in defining and treating it better. They have identified the cause of many previously mysterious pain problems as trigger points. If you could examine a trigger point you would feel it as a nodule or "taut band" in the muscle. Because it actually can cause shortening of the muscle, when you pressed it you might feel the muscle twitch. (This twitch response can be far stronger if the trigger point is stimulated by a needle.)

There are also numerous TrPs in the muscles of the abdomen. These can mimic pain of the contents of the abdomen ("viscera"), and some think they can even induce visceral dysfunction, including some symptoms of Irritable Bowel Syndrome (IBS) and irritable bladder.

Abdominal TrPs are almost always aggravated by movement which would contract the involved muscles such as bending over and lifting. Sometimes the patient may have a bloated abdomen that he cannot "suck in" very well, because contraction of the muscles is inhibited by TrPs. They can also be activated by trauma or mechanical stress which puts a strain on them. Sit-ups, bending over, straining at stool, emotional tension, twisting movements, and leaning over a desk are common precipitants.

The rectus abdominis muscles are situated like two straps that go from the ribs to the pubic bone on either side of the navel. TrPs in these muscles refer pain to organs which are underneath them. Gallbladder pain, non-ulcer dyspepsia (NUD), intestinal spasms, bladder pain, pseudoappendicitis, and menstrual cramps can all be mimicked or caused by TrPs in the relevant area of the rectus abdominis. To further complicate matters, pain originating in the viscera can cause TrPs in the muscles of the torso.

**TREATING TRIGGER POINTS**  Unlike treatments for other illnesses, that for trigger points involves not so much drugs as physical manipulation of the trigger point. For example, a shortened muscle may be maintaining a trigger point. Relieving that muscle by stretching it might also relieve the trigger point and the referred pain. Although it sounds painful—it really isn't too bad—putting needles into the muscle as is done in acupuncture can also relieve the trigger point and remove the pain.

But the most effective treatment is injecting a substance directly into the trigger point. (Not very long ago injections directly into muscles to alleviate trigger points were either unheard of or regarded as quackery. Today they are common.) The results can be amazing and instantaneous, relieving pain not only at the trigger point but at the distant referred-pain site as well. Your doctor should stretch the muscle after the injection to relieve the muscle shortening that helps to maintain the trigger point.

A physician well versed in treating trigger points by injection is the best one to see. The pain can be made considerably worse, not better, if the doctor misses the trigger point. Also, if the problem is not trigger points but tender points (as in fibromyalgia), the pain can also be worsened if they are injected.

I believe that an injection relieves a trigger point by interrupting a complex pathway between the muscle and the spinal cord. Once interrupted, the cause of the pain is gone, although it may return unless precipitating factors such as poor posture are corrected or repetitive activities that strain a muscle are stopped.

## SPECIFIC PAIN AREAS

Thus far we've been talking in general about localized pain and pain syndromes. Now, let's switch gears and talk about three specific kinds of pain that may not be treated properly:

Pain from being immobile
Pain from an operation
Lower back pain

**TRAUMA OR IMMOBILITY PAIN** If you've had an accident and are forced to be immobilized in bed for a period of time, you are at risk to develop a different kind of pain that can be permanent. This pain can occur in an arm or a leg that has been in a cast. It is characterized by burning pain and perspiration in the affected area and involves the beginning of a loss of mineral in the bones. It can also occur after an injury in which nerves are damaged.

Unfortunately, this condition (called reflex sympathetic dystrophy) is often missed early, when it is very treatable with nerve blocks. If your doctor does not diagnose it and it is allowed to progress too long without appropriate treatment, the disorder may become permanent and extremely distressing.

Some of the worst situations occur after orthopedic or podiatric surgery for a painful condition. You may go in for surgery because your foot is giving you a lot of pain. Afterward, when your foot is in a cast, the pain may seem to be getting better. But then, particularly when the cast is removed, the pain may become far worse. The problem is not your original pain site, but nerve damage caused by your foot being in a cast.

By not diagnosing and treating the reflex sympathetic dystrophy, your physician may compound the problem by a well-meaning but mistaken belief that the original painful site was not completely removed. He or she may suggest another operation without realizing that the problem you now have was caused by the immobility resulting from the first surgery.

**POSTOPERATIVE PAIN** There are numerous ways to decrease pain after surgery. Nerve blocks have already been mentioned. One of the newer methods is a technique that allows you to regulate the amount of a pain-suppressing drug entering your body. With patient-controlled analgesia you control intravenous pain medication by pushing a button. (A computer makes sure you don't get too much all at once or cumulatively, which could be harmful.)

Patients who use this technique require less pain medication and report less discomfort than those who traditionally have waited for the overworked nurse to get around to giving them a "pain shot." Pain can be relieved much more easily when it is just beginning than when it is very severe.

Some surgeons still do not know how to prescribe patient-controlled pain medication or are worried that patients might become addicted during their three to five postoperative days. However, addiction to narcotics in a hospital setting usually takes much longer.

**LOWER BACK PAIN**  An enormous amount has been written about lower back pain, and it is beyond the scope of this book to deal with all aspects. We shall restrict ourselves to two frequently overlooked or misdiagnosed areas. (Such causes of lower back pain as cancer and herniated discs are not discussed here. If you have chronic or recurrent back pain you should have a complete work-up by an orthopedist to be sure of the cause.)

**Trigger Points in Lower Back Pain**  Most of my patients who complain of a "wrenched back" have trigger points in the hollow spots where the spine joins the pelvis. More often than not I can relieve this pain rapidly with an injection of a salt solution (normal saline) into the trigger point.

I have done this thousands of times and have never had a complication. If it works, the pain is gone almost immediately. This trigger-point injection is not very painful, either. Since acute lower back pain is so common, very primary-care doctor should know how to do this procedure.

**Pelvic Muscles in Lower Back Pain**  One of the pelvic muscles can cause lower back pain and abdominal pain (as well as painful intercourse for women). This muscle (the pyriformis) can cause a condition that can be confused with sciatica or lower back nerve pain. Occasionally I see a patient who has had one or more back surgeries for supposed disc problems, but the pain remains. When this happens the poor patient is placed in the unfortunate category of "failed back syndrome," which is even worse than it sounds.

Fortunately, sometimes the pain is actually part of a my-ofascial syndrome and can be easily treated. A pelvic muscle pain syndrome is more common in women than in men, prob-ably because of the shape of the pelvis, and is sometimes seen after the affected muscles have been shortened for a period of time, as when the legs are spread during a vaginal hys-terectomy.

Your doctor should be able to diagnose this problem easily. To do so, he presses the pyriform muscle either rectally or vaginally. The muscle will be exquisitely tender if it is the cause of the pain. If this is the case, the affected muscle can be treated like any other trigger point: by injection with normal saline. Often pain and accompanying numbness, which may go down into the leg, are instantly relieved.

The injection itself can be a bit painful, but the results are often worth it. The doctor may inject through the buttocks, while pressing on the muscle with his finger in the rectum or through the vagina so he knows where to aim the needle. A "caudal" block, an injection of local anesthetic and a corti-sone derivative, may also be given around the lower spinal nerves.

Do not count on your gynecologist to discover this problem automatically. Gynecologists do not usually press the muscles of the pelvic floor when doing a pelvic exam, even when they are looking for causes of pelvic pain (other pelvic muscles may be involved also), and often miss this easily diagnosable con-dition.

**Exercise for Lower Back Pain** Another remedy for lower back pain is exercise, which is very important in order to reduce pain and prevent its recurrence. All sorts of exercises are available but I always suggest two, both of which involve muscle stretching and trigger-point inactivation. Both exercises are done lying on your back. (Check with your doctor first to be sure you don't have a more serious back problem such as a severely herniated disc, which could preclude doing these exercises.)

**Exercise One: Stretching the Hamstrings.** The ham-strings are the muscles in the back of the thigh. Raise your legs up, one at a time, until perpendicular with your body. Do this ten to twenty times a day. If your hamstrings are tight you will not be able to get your legs up this high right away, but you will in a few weeks.

**Exercise Two: Knee Bend.**    Lie on your back, bend one knee, put the other leg over it, and push down on the bottom leg until the inside part of the knee touches the floor. Hold it there for five seconds. Repeat this on both sides five to ten times a day. This exercise stretches the buttock muscles, and you will often feel your back pop as if you have just visited a chiropractor.

You will probably not be able to push your knee to the floor at first, but in a few weeks it should be fairly easy. By that time you may wonder how you ever survived before without doing these and other exercises regularly.

## THE PAIN THAT ISN'T THERE
### (CHRONIC INTRACTABLE BENIGN PAIN)

Patients with chronic intractable benign pain may go to their doctor's office complaining bitterly. However, the doctor who finds nothing apparently wrong, not even tender points or trigger points, may say "It's all in your head!" (the not-uncommon diagnosis for many mysterious maladies).

In pain clinics this diagnosis is called chronic intractable benign pain or somatoform pain disorder. Clinically "The essential feature of this disorder is preoccupation with pain in the absence of adequate physical findings to account for the pain or its intensity" (in the words of *DSM-III-R*, the diagnostic manual for psychiatric disorders).

Maybe the pain *is* in your head and maybe psychological counseling is necessary (see Chapter 13). But before resigning yourself to this, be sure that your exam was thorough.

It's especially important to ensure that your physician knows about fibromyalgia and myofascial pain syndrome and that you have been examined for these disorders. It would be a mistake automatically to assume that he has. Don't feel embarrassed to ask if your doctor has expertise in this area. Remember, you are a partner in your health care.

Many physicians still do not believe that fibromyalgia exists, despite enormous evidence to the contrary and numerous publications in highly regarded medical journals. Prior to the late 1970s most doctors had never heard of a trigger point. Of those who have now heard of them, many still do not know how to examine for trigger points.

In short, be aware that the absence of physical findings could be due to the absence of knowledge on the part of the examining physician about fibromyalgia and myofascial pain syndrome and not to some mental illness on your part. (Some of my patients with pain diagnosed as in their heads were never examined systematically for trigger points and hence their fibromyalgia or myofascial pain syndrome was overlooked.)*

If, however, you do have pain when there truly is no physical cause, psychological counseling as well as the comprehensive approach to pain management that can be found in a pain clinic is in order.

## SEVERE PAIN FROM AN INCURABLE DISEASE

Thus far we've talked about "benign" pain. Now we consider a different class of pain, that caused by cancer.

**CANCER PAIN**  The cause of cancer pain is usually obvious but may not be curable. Cancer can produce severe pain, since the disease can change the structure of the body. In the past even morphine injections were not fully effective against such pain. The patient was left to suffer, often horribly, for extended periods. Today there are effective ways to treat cancer pain. With epidural (meaning around the coverings of the spinal cord) analgesia, pain-relieving chemicals of various sorts (usually morphine or a related substance) are infused continuously by a computerized container implanted under the skin.

*I am not alone in this discovery. Experience similar to mine was described by H. Rosomoff and others in an article "Physical findings in patients with chronic intractable benign pain of the neck and/or back," *Pain*, vol. 37 (1989), pp. 279–287. Thirty-four patients with neck pain and ninety patients with lower back pain who fit the criteria for benign pain were all found to have signs of myofascial pain syndrome and/or fibromyalgia. Some of Rosomoff's patients were actually thought to have hysterical disorders because their pain, and sometimes numbness, radiated to different areas of their body. Even though this symptom is characteristic of trigger points, in these cases the initial examining physicians were not aware of trigger points or related illnesses and did not diagnose them. This unfortunate situation is probably quite common.

Another technique is to inject pain-producing nerves with substances that destroy them. A good example of this procedure is the celiac plexus block. Here pancreatic pain, from either cancer or inflammation of the pancreas, is alleviated by destroying the nerve cells that produce the pain. The nerve bundle that goes to the pancreas (among other organs) is first injected with a local anesthetic. If the pain is relieved temporarily, this nerve bundle is the cause. Then it is reinjected with a material that destroys it. Destroying the nerves transmitting the pain does not cure the illness, but it does help make the patient far more comfortable.

## UNTREATABLE CHRONIC PAIN

What to do for the patient with chronic pain not due to cancer who is untreatable by the types of techniques we have discussed?

One option could be having a doctor prescribe opioid (narcoticlike) medication. Most physicians are understandably reluctant to do this on an extended basis because of the realistic concern for addiction. (Recent articles in the medical literature, however, suggest that abuse does not take place in the pain patient who does not already abuse other drugs.) For the physician who is still reluctant, I would suggest a group of narcoticlike drugs that not only relieve pain but may also cause unpleasant reactions. The more you take, the more unpleasant you feel, and hence the less likely you are to abuse the substance.

Another option is one of the drugs below, some of the many now available for untreatable chronic pain. It might be necessary for you and your physician to consider the following drugs.

A new injectable NSAID (nonsteroid anti-inflammatory drug), ketorolac (Toradal), reputed to be as potent as morphine, is not addicting at all and is available by prescription.

Buprenorphine (Buprenex) is an injectable narcotic with supposedly lowered addiction potential. In other countries it is available in a form taken under the tongue that is reported to be just as potent as taking it by injection. Buprenex may also have the surprising ability to block the symptoms of withdrawal from cocaine.

Other similar medications work in unusual ways. Weak enzyme inhibitors such as enalapril (Vasotec), captopril (Capoten), and lisinopril (Prinivil, Zestril)—drugs used to reduce high blood pressure—may raise the levels of morphinelike substances naturally produced by the body by inhibiting the enzymes that destroy them. Some patients are quite sensitive to their beneficial enzyme-inhibiting effects; many have told me their pain lessens when they take them. Tolerance does not seem to develop with these drugs.

Many other substances in the body affect pain; calcitonin is one of them. It has been primarily used lately in treating osteoporosis but has been reported to relieve certain kinds of pain involving abnormal nerve transmission, especially after amputation, when the patient still feels his painful limb even though it is not there.

Octreotide (Somatostatin), used normally to combat diarrhea, may be able to treat many kinds of pain.

Clonidine, used for high blood pressure and given epidurally (near the spine), may produce pain relief for up to a month, although it may cause a drop in blood pressure.

Experimental narcotics that do not appear to be habit-forming may soon be available. This claim has been made for other narcotic pain-killers that could be addictive or abused in more widespread use. Perhaps that will not be the case with these newer agents. Ask your doctor about them. One is named tramadol.

Remember that these are all prescription medications. Discuss each with your physician: It may be that one or all are not appropriate. On the other hand, one or more may help relieve your pain.

**CHANGING YOUR MENTAL OUTLOOK**   Finally, there is the matter of living with pain. Some outstanding pain specialists believe that any pain can be treated by altering the way you understand it and deal with it emotionally. This method gives you some control over your pain and allows you to live a more effective and satisfying life despite it. Family participation that uses cognitive-behavioral therapy (discussed in more detail in Chapter 13), is an important part of this approach.

While results have been reported to be very good and I do

not disagree with this assessment for the most part, I have seen patients who have not done well. In short, I do not favor this treatment used alone except as a last resort.

There are two reasons for problems with cognitive-behavioral therapy. First, there may be over-reliance on it as the primary treatment. This is terribly damaging if you were originally misdiagnosed. You and your doctor should try to eliminate the cause of the pain and exhaust all diagnostic methods before resorting to cognitive-behavioral therapy.

The second reason cognitive-behavioral therapy may be ineffective is that you may not be able to afford it (or be able to afford it the number of times or in the setting it requires; much chronic-pain therapy of this kind must be done in a hospital). Many patients who are advised to seek chronic-pain therapy either have exhausted their insurance coverage, have no insurance, or the insurance carrier will not pay for this service since it is regarded as psychiatric treatment and health insurance often pays for psychiatric treatment at a lower rate.

If your doctor is still mystified about the cause of your pain, you might suggest a technique called a "differential spinal block" that may help in diagnosis. This procedure, which will only block nerves below the waist, can be quite informative.

If pain is still present when the affected part is numb—as evidenced, for example, by your being unable to move your legs—it is undoubtedly central pain. In other words, this pain comes not from the extremities but from the brain and may indeed be treatable by cognitive-behavioral therapy. On the other hand, if the pain is eliminated by differential spinal block, it does come from the legs and therefore might be more effectively treated by one of the methods detailed above.

This diagnostic technique has pitfalls in cases in which the pain could be referred. But a tip-off for your doctor that you may have central pain is that your pain may actually increase when nerve transmission is blocked. Even central pain can be treated by medications which increase the amount of the neurotransmitter acetylcholine in the brain. Antidepressants are frequently used. In the future other agents will doubtless also be found effective.

## READING MORE ABOUT PAIN MEDICINE

We've only scratched the surface of the variety of techniques available to reduce pain.

If you would like to investigate the topic of pain medicine further, try *Textbook of Pain* (2nd edition), edited by Patrick D. Wall and Ronald Melzack (New York: Churchill Livingstone, 1989). This book is a bit deep for the average reader but it contains much valuable information.

For more about trigger points and commonly misdiagnosed pain problems that involve the muscles, look into the quite-readable *Myofascial Pain and Dysfunction: The Trigger-Point Manual* by Janet G. Travell and David G. Simons (Baltimore: Williams & Wilkins, 1983). This book is one of the most useful I have read on the subject although it only deals with pain in the upper half of the body. (A second volume will deal with the lower half.)

# 2

## Sleep Disorders

Ideally I would first explain why we sleep. Unfortunately, I can't; no one knows why! That's right, after twenty or thirty years of intensive research efforts, the basic function of sleep is still not understood. No one knows why we dream, either. Sleep is nevertheless an essential part of existence; virtually all creatures sleep at one time or another and many also dream.

The fact that we don't know why we sleep does not mean, however, that we know nothing about it. In recent years many sleep disorders have been discovered. Perhaps the one most recently discussed is sleep apnea, a condition in which the sleeper actually stops breathing as many as five hundred times during a night and that can be fatal.

Other sleep disorders include snoring, which, associated with sleep apnea, can be a serious problem. There are also narcolepsy (the victim falls asleep during the day) and insomnia (he or she can't fall asleep during the night).

Doctors are becoming increasingly aware of sleep disorders, but many patients still do not get their problems correctly diagnosed or treated. In fact, the diagnosis of disordered sleep is one of the general disciplines of medicine in which I believe physicians are the most poorly trained. Too often you may see your doctor with a complaint of insomnia, for example, and be given sleeping pills. Or your snoring may be dismissed simply as a humorous but not serious malady. These approaches are inappropriate.

31

## WHAT HAPPENS WHEN YOU SLEEP

There are two distinct phases to sleep:

- Rapid eye movement (REM). Sleep in which the eyes go back and forth under closed eyelids.
- Non-REM (NREM) sleep. Four separate stages that are characterized by how deeply a person is sleeping and measured by brain-wave pattern seen on an EEG. These patterns are graded from Stage I to Stage IV.

**GOING TO SLEEP**   We begin sleep with the non-REM phase and then alternate with REM sleep during the night; the first NREM period usually lasts sixty to ninety minutes. As sleep progresses we have less non-REM sleep and more REM sleep, with about 75 percent non-REM in one of its lighter stages.

**WHILE WE SLEEP**   While we sleep we dream. Dreaming typically occurs during REM sleep, although not all REM sleep is dreaming. When we dream during REM, our moving eyes appear to be looking at things. Our inner ears also seem to be activated, perhaps sensing motion.

**CHARACTERISTICS OF SLEEP**   A number of unusual characteristics of REM and non-REM sleep are quite distinct and also help to define them for us. For example, we have near-paralysis of our voluntary muscles during REM sleep, and some disorders are caused by a failure of this paralysis during sleep. During REM sleep we are also sensitive to temperature changes.

During NREM sleep we do not have formed dreams, but are also not paralyzed—our involuntary muscles are no longer inhibited—and we are not sensitive to temperature changes.

Most sleep disorders are associated with unusual REM sleep or the suppression of REM and/or NREM sleep or the fragmentation of sleep with frequent awakenings (sometimes as often as hundreds of times), even though we do not remember them in the morning except for feeling sleepy.

**SLEEP RHYTHMS**   The time we sleep is closely related to certain biological rhythms (circadian rhythms). These rhythms cause us to tend to fall asleep at the same time each night and wake about the same time each morning. Breaking these rhythms, as when we travel across time zones or shift our working pattern, can cause insomnia at night and excessive sleepiness during the day.

## NARCOLEPSY

Narcolepsy, one of the earliest sleep disorders to be medically described, is generally thought to be an intrusion of REM sleep into normal wakefulness, causing the victim to fall asleep when he or she should be awake.

The four classic symptoms of narcolepsy are:

**1. Virtually irresistible daytime sleep attacks**   These last from a few minutes to an hour, resulting in a feeling of refreshment and may recur throughout the day. Many physicians do not understand that the urge to sleep is overpowering.

**2. Loss of muscle control (cataplexy)**   Cataplexy causes total loss of motor control so that the narcoleptic falls and is essentially paralyzed for a brief time. This phenomenon generally occurs during periods of emotion, such as when laughing or sad, but can also occur during increased fatigue.
Diagnosis of this symptom in its classical state is quite easy, and most physicians won't confuse it with any other illness except a kind of epilepsy called akinetic seizures.

The doctor may have trouble diagnosing it, however, when it is not full-blown, which is usually the case. Here there is not total inhibition of all the muscles, only of isolated muscle groups. As a result your legs may buckle unexpectedly, causing you to fall, or you may drop things for no reason at all. Afterward, you may feel generally weak for a while but not fall down.

Other muscle groups may be involved in numerous ways. The attack may be preceded by only very mild emotion and may not suggest cataplexy to the physician. Although attacks may last up to half an hour, often they last for only a few seconds.

This momentary loss of muscle control can bewilder the patient. And because they really don't realize they've just had a ''sleep attack,'' they can't effectively describe what happened. As a result, the condition is often ignored by many physicians or incorrectly diagnosed as a nerve problem or perhaps a small stroke. It can be correctly diagnosed by a device that measures muscle function, an electromyogram (EMG), that can be worn during daily activities.

**3. Sleep paralysis** In this condition one is unable to move, usually at the onset of sleep but also on awakening. It can occur briefly in normal people, but in narcoleptics it can last as long as ten minutes and can be quite frightening. It is often accompanied by hallucinations.

Sleep paralysis and hallucinations can be very mild, seeming not to occur at all. Several years may pass after the onset of narcoleptic attacks before it becomes evident.

When you describe this problem your physician may refer you to a psychiatrist. Many doctors are unfamiliar with the symptoms of narcolepsy, and sleep paralysis is often one that is misunderstood. Don't let it be ignored: It can be treated.

**4. Hallucinations** These occur at the same time as sleep paralysis. Usually visual, they can also be auditory or tactile. They may be unformed if visual, but also may involve persons or animals who act in an unusual way. Occasionally they may be unpleasant or threatening. They may seem more like projections on a movie screen than a dream.

**PROBLEMS IN DIAGNOSING NARCOLEPSY** Unless you have typical narcolepsy, many physicians will misdiagnose your problem. Daytime sleep attacks will be confused with simple fatigue. Temporary loss of muscle control may bring neurological explanations, such as seizures, hysteria, or multiple sclerosis. The same can be true of sleep paralysis, although hysteria might be more commonly diagnosed.

A good doctor, however, will add up all the symptoms and come to the right conclusion. To confirm it he may ask you to take a test called the Multiple Sleep Latency Test (MSLT). You will first be evaluated in a sleep laboratory with a number of measures (polysomnography) to make sure you do not have some other sleep disorder, such as sleep apnea, that could also cause excessive daytime sleepiness. You will also be evaluated to see whether you are suffering from lack of REM sleep during the preceding night that needs to be made up for. Once other problems are ruled out, you will be asked to take sequential daytime naps at two-hour intervals. If you fall asleep rapidly and have REM sleep right away (sleep normally begins with non-REM sleep), the diagnosis of narcolepsy is established.

Another test for narcolepsy is a blood test called HLA-DR2 for a genetic marker that is frequently present in narcoleptics. (A few narcoleptics have other unusual diseases that may have a genetic component as well.)

**GETTING THE RIGHT TREATMENTS**    Treatments for narcolepsy usually involve drug therapy with effective drugs, usually stimulants, such as methylphenidate (Ritalin).

Treatment of narcolepsy has been greatly aided by testing on a group of genetically narcoleptic dogs at Stanford University. These dogs have increased levels of a chemical called acetylcholine, which induces REM sleep. Therefore stimulants and compounds that block acetylcholine have been used to treat the disorders-of-excessive-daytime-sleepiness (described later in this chapter) aspect of narcolepsy. Sometimes I prescribe protriptylene (Vivactil) for all aspects of narcolepsy because of its stimulating effects. Vivactil is generally used as an antidepressant.

Narcoleptics can also take naps during the day when convenient, since, for a period of time after a nap, sleep attacks will not occur.

**PROBLEMS WITH TREATMENT**    Your doctor may be skeptical if you walk in and claim to be narcoleptic, at least at first. The drugs used in treatment are often the sort that can be abused.

Doctors are sometimes faced with someone who isn't narcoleptic but is a drug abuser who wants a prescription for Dexedrine (an ''upper''). Your physician may have treated such patients, prescribed the drug, then never saw them again. For this reason most physicians will insist that a patient who has narcoleptic symptoms have an MSLT so that the diagnosis can be as certain as possible.

But narcoleptics are not necessarily drug abusers. Also, a

new drug—an antidepressant not yet available in the United States—called viloxazine treats all aspects of narcolepsy, is nonaddictive, and is not a controlled substance which can cause problems for doctors.

**INSURANCE PROBLEMS WITH NARCOLEPSY**    Health insurance often will not pay for polysomnography or MSLTs. Testing for sleep disorders is expensive. And, because of the cost, some health maintenance organizations (HMOs) do not have the facilities.

## INSOMNIA

From a medical viewpoint, insomnia is a condition in which sleep is disturbed and, as a result, a person does not feel he or she has slept enough. Most people who complain of insomnia do, indeed, have some form of disturbed sleep. (A subtype of patients called pseudoinsomniacs actually do have sleep of normal length and normal sleep architecture (the timing and distribution of REM and NREM sleep) but persist in saying and feeling that they have not slept well.)

Although we all have it occasionally, for a large minority of the population insomnia is a significant problem. Close to 15 percent of the population regard insomnia as a problem that diminishes the quality of their lives.

**PROBLEMS IN DEALING WITH INSOMNIA**    Two essential problems are involved with insomnia: (1) the inability to fall asleep when you want to and the resulting feelings of tiredness and (2) the use of sleeping pills by insomniacs. Generally these pills do not cure the insomnia and in many cases may make it chronic by causing the patient to become addicted to them. As we'll see, there are ways of handling insomnia that do not involve popping sleeping pills.

**TRANSIENT INSOMNIA**    Transient insomnia is very common; almost everyone experiences it at one time or another. It is usually related to stress and is time-limited, lasting a maximum of two to three weeks. Although this type of insomnia is fairly benign, if you do not have it treated properly, it may convert to longer-lasting disorders.

Besides stress, common causes of transient insomnia are jet lag, and a somewhat similar situation, shiftwork on the grave-yard or swing shift. In both cases you are asked to sleep at a time different from what you are accustomed to, and as a re-sult, you usually experience difficulty falling and staying asleep.

Transient stress-related insomnia is the major reason doctors prescribe sleeping pills, which are usually a short-acting form of a drug class called benzodiazepines. If you do take them, they probably won't be addictive if you take them for less than three weeks. They should only be used as a temporary aid. If for some reason you are required to take them longer, you should take them intermittently to minimize habituation and tolerance to their effects.

Keep in mind that the real problem with transient insomnia is sleep habits that need to be straightened out.

**Circadian Rhythms** In order to better understand the problems of transient insomnia—specifically of jet lag and shiftwork—as well as how to correct them, we need first to talk about the biological rhythms of the body. These biological rhythms are organized around roughly a twenty-four-hour pe-riod and are called circadian (from the Latin *circa*-approximately, *dies*-day). Most other processes in the body—mental alertness, hormone secretion, antibiotic sensitivity, and so on—rise and fall to their own rhythms, usually at different times of the day.

Circadian rhythms are generated by structures inside the brain in a very important region called the hypothalamus. They are also influenced by external cues such as light and dark, work and leisure, and other regular events. The details of cir-cadian physiology are very complex and a rapidly expanding research specialty.

So far as insomnia is concerned, the circadian rhythms tell us when to be awake and when to fall asleep. But sometimes we get "out of phase." Then we feel very alert when we should be sleeping and very sleepy when we should be alert, generally a short-lived problem. However, if it lasts more than six months it is considered a serious sleep phase disorder.

A common cause of transient insomnia is the delayed sleep phase syndrome. You cannot fall asleep until the early morning hours, just before you must get up for work. Waking up is difficult because you just fell asleep, and you feel sleep-deprived. The sleep itself is usually normal and you will feel rested if allowed to sleep your desired period (usually seven to eight hours).

Beware of doctors who without a thorough diagnosis suggest you have depression or anxiety when you complain of transient insomnia. In either of these disorders, patients have abnormal and disrupted sleep. In transient insomnia, the sleep itself is normal.

**Treating Delayed Sleep Phase Syndrome**   Usually the best treatment is to take a vacation. During your vacation stress should be relieved. In addition, you should get yourself back on the correct circadian cycle: Go to bed three hours later each night until you arrive at the time you would like to go to sleep and then stay there. Napping is not allowed.

A more drastic approach, faster but not as effective, is to not sleep at all for twenty-four hours and then go to bed at the desired time.

There are other variations on this theme. For example, you may get a full eight hours of sleep in one twenty-four-hour period, but you must do it in two or more sleep periods instead of all at once.

Above all, you must stop napping. It will take a while, but eventually you should be able retrain yourself to a single seven-to-eight-hour sleep cycle.

**Jet Lag**   There are various strategies for dealing with jet lag, none of them entirely satisfactory. Generally speaking, whatever you do requires one day per hour of time change to readjust the biological clock, especially when flying eastward. In other words, if you fly from California to New York, it will take you three days to adjust fully. Recent research suggests that being in bright light at some point during the day can shorten that time.

**Shiftwork**   Insomnia due to shiftwork is more difficult to resolve, since people who work the evening and (especially) the night shifts do not have the usual environmental cues such as light and dark and social interactions to readjust their sleep–wake cycles.

Current wisdom holds that if you are going to work on a swing or graveyard shift, don't do it just for a short time. Shift changes should last longer than one week in order for your body to adapt. Furthermore, they should progress from day to evening to night. (If your supervisors don't understand this, show them this book. They should recognize that violating these principles can result in an increased error rate, more employee sick time, and lowered performance.) During the first week, when you are adjusting, demands should be minimized since you simply won't be able to perform up to par. Sleeping pills may be used effectively for the first day or two after a shift change.

A recent discovery is that bright light itself can affect the shift work. As reported in the *New England Journal of Medicine,* volunteers who worked at night responded very well when their workplace was brightly lighted and when, after work, they went to sleep in a totally dark room. The report (by Dr. Charles A. Czeisler and others) suggests that the body's rhythms respond very quickly to light and so, by mimicking natural light and dark at the opposite times of the twenty-four-hour cycle, we can convince the body to be awake during the night and asleep during the day.

**Primary Insomnia** Beyond stress, jet lag, and shiftwork, we come to primary insomnia. *Primary* here does not mean "first"; it means that psychiatric disorders are not thought to be the cause. Primary insomnia is thought to be due to worry, poor coping mechanisms for stress, and difficulty in relaxing.

If you have primary insomnia you may have trouble falling asleep and (if it is severe) decreased REM sleep with frequent awakening. Primary insomnia is usually viewed as a "learned" disorder. By this I mean that if you go to bed and, instead of falling asleep, you ruminate on how your life is going or about what happened during the day, you're learning to stay awake. If you wonder about whether or not you will have trouble falling asleep you usually do.

Since almost everyone at one time or another has had insomnia induced by the stresses of daily life, the reason only certain people develop primary insomnia is not actually known, but it can be seen as a problem of the "tuning" of your nervous-system control. The arousal system of the brain in primary insomniacs may be tuned higher than in most people. In other words, it takes less to awaken you and keep you awake.

Another possible cause of primary insomnia could be excessive stimulant use. While stimulants could mean amphetamines or cocaine, coffee, which many people drink habitually at work, is often the special culprit. If you take coffee as a drug and use it to maintain alertness, the coffee itself may continue keeping you awake at night. Reducing (or, better still, eliminating) the coffee may cure your insomnia. The sleep disturbing effects of a cup of coffee can last up to eight hours.

Another cause may be generalized anxiety disorder, discussed in Chapter 13. People with generalized anxiety disorder are worried and fearful about many aspects of their lives. Nevertheless, patients with primary insomnia focus primarily on sleep as their big problem.

**Treating Primary Insomnia**  Sleeping pills should not be used to treat primary insomnia. If they are used, they should be taken only under unusual circumstances, once or twice a month. If your doctor prescribes sleeping pills for this condition, it's time to seek other medical advice.

The easiest way to treat primary insomnia can be to alter your conditioning. For example, use the bedroom only for sex and sleep. When going to sleep, do not go into the bedroom unless you feel sleepy. If you are not asleep within ten minutes, leave the bedroom. Go somewhere else in the house and engage in some relaxing activity until you feel sleepy, then go back to bed.

Alcohol in excess of one or two ounces should not be consumed near bedtime as a sleep inducer. When alcohol is metabolized, you have a miniwithdrawal reaction and often suddenly awaken perspiring and hot, with a rapid heart rate. This makes it difficult to go back to sleep and further conditions you to worry about your sleep problem unless you're already aware of this effect of alcohol. Cigarette smoking may also delay sleep onset, since nicotine releases adrenalin from the adrenal glands.

**LIFELONG INSOMNIA**  Some people have never been able to sleep well, even as children. I knew a fellow in college who seemed to be constantly up. Over several years I don't think

I ever saw him sleep more than two or three times and then only for short periods. When I asked him if he was tired, he almost invariably said yes. When I asked why he didn't, then, lie down and go to sleep, he said he simply couldn't. This condition typically starts in childhood and lasts the rest of one's life.

People with lifelong insomnia usually have a congenital defect in their neurological sleep circuitry. They may also have abnormal sleep. Other problems may also be present, such as attention deficit disorder with hyperactivity (see Chapter 14).

Of course, lifelong insomnia does not necessarily occur with the same degree of severity all the time. It may wax and wane. Sometimes it is a more severe version of primary insomnia and occurs on a continuum where virtually no stress to quite severe stress might be required to trigger it. The amount of stress required may vary according to an individual's genetic susceptibility.

Most people who have this disorder are resigned to living with it. They know that sleeping pills can be highly addictive if they are taken over long periods of time and tend to avoid them.

There are things, however, which can help. Adjusting sleep habits are helpful but usually do not cure the problem. Useful treatment may involve long-term use of sedating medications such as doxepin (Sinequan), amitriptyline (Elavil), or trazodone (Desyrel). Occasionally I use low doses of thioridazine (Mellaril) as well.

**DISORDERS OF INITIATING AND MAINTAINING SLEEP** If you have this sleep disorder, not only do you have trouble falling asleep but, once asleep, you tend to wake up repeatedly.

A problem may arise if your doctor wants to treat this problem as though it were transient insomnia caused by stress or jet lag or shiftwork. In other words, he may ask you to take a few sleeping pills until it goes away.

Unfortunately, this approach usually doesn't work because this disorder is usually a symptom of underlying psychological problems. Counseling may be in order, since proper treatment involves resolving these underlying problems. Then the sleep disorder usually disappears.

In addition, many physical problems that cause pain or discomfort can also cause this difficulty. If you have trouble falling asleep and staying asleep, you should have a thorough medical evaluation to see if medical problems are present and then treat them as effectively as possible.

A disorder of initiating and maintaining sleep is also the most common sleep disorder seen in patients with Chronic Fatigue Syndrome, who frequently complain that they cannot fall asleep even though they are so exhausted they can hardly move. Then, once asleep, they wake up. (Since lack of sleep can make CFS much worse, treating the disorder in Chronic Fatigue Syndrome has a very high priority.)


## SNORING

Snoring has its humorous side and thus is sometimes ignored medically. However, snoring can be associated with serious disorders and should never be taken lightly.

Snoring is caused by a reduction of muscle tension in the tongue and throat muscles. When you breathe in while sleeping, the force of the air going down the windpipe causes the muscles of the throat to vibrate because they are being pulled downward and closer together. As air goes by them the vibrations produce sound, somewhat like playing a wind instrument. The danger is that if the muscles come too close together, air cannot get through and breathing stops. I sometimes compare this to sucking too hard on a straw. If you suck too hard, the straw collapses.

Snoring occurs most often when you lie on your back. (An old remedy was to sew a tennis ball into the back of your pajamas so you can't lie that way.) When you're on your back, your tongue falls more into your throat, because of gravity, than when you sleep in some other position.

Snoring can also be caused by sedative drugs. Some people have narrower airways than others. Others have a genetic predisposition to snore.

Snoring is very common. More men snore than do women, and it occurs more in obese people than those of normal weight. And the incidence of snoring increases with age.

Snoring can sometimes be so loud that it can be heard throughout an entire house, and occasionally in neighboring houses. It can even exceed the standards of safe levels of sound exposure! Snoring can even take its toll on marriages; the sleep-deprived spouse of a snorer can be quite irritable.

**DANGERS OF SNORING** In the 1960s it was realized that snoring was associated with sleep apnea. Since sleep apnea has achieved so much notoriety (see the next section), doctors have begun to be careful about dismissing snoring out of hand. But still, if you snore, one problem is finding a doctor who will take your snoring seriously. Many physicians still ignore it. Relatively few doctors recognize that recent research indicates that snoring is related to high blood pressure and possibly decreased blood flow to the heart and brain.

The second biggest problem tends to be treatment. Those who do take snoring seriously may want you to rush off and have surgery. While surgery can be successful, in many cases it is not. It often involves removing the uvula (the little tag of skin that hangs down at the back of the mouth), the adenoids and tonsils, and even part of the palate. The result can be that fluids you drink inadvertently come out of your nose. Some patients also report that after surgery the timbre of their voices becomes more nasal.

**TREATING SNORING** Rather than begin with surgery, the easiest way to treat snoring is to lose weight. The reason obesity causes snoring and sleep apnea is not clear, although it is assumed that fatty deposits in the airway further narrows it. While this has not been clearly shown, often the loss of only ten or fifteen pounds will significantly reduce your snoring.

Drugs of various sorts have also been tried to treat snoring, and the conventional wisdom is that they either do not work or the adverse reactions associated with them are too great. I have not found this to be the case in the many snorers I have treated with protriptylene (Vivactil). This drug tends to increase the nerve activity of the nerves that go to the muscles of the airway, the very ones that have decreased tone and that relax too much when snorers sleep. With this medication the increased nerve activity increases the muscle tone and snoring often decreases or stops. In my experience, snoring often decreases with as little as 2.5 mg. Vivactil daily; and the highest I have prescribed is 10 mg. At these doses, not many patients have complained of intolerance, and many of their spouses have been extremely grateful.

While Vivactil treatment is worth a try, it does not work very well when the airway collapse is severe enough to obstruct breathing. I always encourage my patients who snore to be checked for sleep apnea.

Many other drugs have been tried in treating snoring and various kinds of sleep apnea, but with little success except in unusual cases. One technique of value can be used if you have a stuffy or runny nose (rhinitis). Since most people tend to breathe through their noses when asleep, the nose problem may contribute to the snoring. In this case decongestants and antihistamines can be helpful. However, if your doctor suggests that you take these, make sure he is not giving you the kind that get into the brain and cause sedation, which can increase snoring. Nasal sprays containing a form of cortisone not absorbed into the body such as beclomethasone (Vancenase, Beconase) and cromolyn (Nasalcrom) may also be used. This type of treatment may be effective if your snoring is not related to anatomic abnormalities of the nose such as a deviated nasal septum.

## SLEEP APNEA

Sleep apnea (which means "without breath" in Latin) is the major focus of sleep medicine today. It is probably the only serious sleep disorder the average person has heard of and may, indeed, be the only sleep disorder besides insomnia that some physicians will diagnose. Even so, sleep apnea remains greatly underdiagnosed. And even though most doctors have a heightened awareness of the condition, they may not question family members about sleep apnea in a patient who snores or complains of excessive sleepiness. They tend to believe that it is relatively rare, which it is not. It is perhaps more common than anyone suspects.

Sleep apnea simply means that you stop breathing while asleep. You may have heard someone who had this problem and did not even realize what it was. Typically the person will be snoring while asleep. If you listen closely you will hear a pause often lasting a half-minute or longer during which the person does not breathe. This may end with a little gasp of air as the sleeper tries to catch up. If you've heard this, you've heard sleep apnea.

The great danger, of course, is that one of the times the

person stops breathing will last so long that oxygen to the brain and heart will be depleted and the person will simply not breathe again. When this happens, sleep apnea can be fatal.

**DIAGNOSING SLEEP APNEA**  Any time a patient comes to me complaining of snoring, I immediately suspect sleep apnea. I then routinely perform tests that involve checking breathing during sleep.

Often the diagnosis of sleep apnea is made by a family member, a husband or wife who notices that the spouse is not breathing for periods of time while asleep. If you notice this and take the problem to your doctor and he shrugs it off without suggesting the appropriate tests to determine if sleep apnea is present, it may be time to consult a new doctor, perhaps a specialist in sleep medicine.

The diagnosis of sleep apnea should determine not only if you have it, but what kind it is. There are three kinds:

*Obstructive,* which usually occurs in snorers and results from an obstruction of the airway

*Central,* which occurs as a result of a problem the brain has in controlling breathing while the person sleeps

*Mixed,* when there is both an obstruction and a central problem

**OBSTRUCTIVE SLEEP APNEA**  This most common kind of sleep apnea is obstructive and is frequently associated with snoring. The classic patient with obstructive sleep apnea is an obese middle-aged male with a red face. When he falls asleep, he snores and jerks around somewhat.

Although few patients I see have all of these characteristics, they do highlight many of the symptoms to watch for and include:

Loud snoring

Abnormal movements during sleep (usually caused by low levels of oxygen)

Choking sensations during the night (which may persist even after awakening because muscle tone in the airways is not immediately regained)

Night sweats

Also, if you have this disorder, it is more common for you to awaken to urinate at night and to have more heartburn than if you do not.

During the day, obstructive sleep apnea patients tend to experience a disorder of excessive sleepiness, a related problem. The reason for this is that during the night they have numerous awakenings in order to get the airway open, which disturb the normal sleep architecture. As a result, they easily fall asleep during many daytime activities, especially relaxing, repetitive, or boring ones.

Other common symptoms of obstructive sleep apnea include problems with memory and concentration and personality changes, with depression and irritability leading the list. Still other symptoms include loss of sexual drive, inability to maintain an erection, and morning headaches.

I have seen almost all of these symptoms in my obstructive sleep apnea patients, enabling me to make the diagnosis on the spot—although it certainly needs to be confirmed by polysomnography. A few people make too much blood (polycythemia), accounting for the classic red face, although sometimes this can actually be a symptom of alcohol abuse. Alcohol, a depressant, makes obstructive sleep apnea worse.

Treating obstructive sleep apnea is similar to treating snoring. An additional very effective technique, widely used in obstructive sleep disorder, is continuous positive airway pressure, in which air is constantly blown into your nose and throat while you sleep. While at first this is uncomfortable, many people get used to it, and it does keep your airway open.

**Central Sleep Apnea**    In central sleep apnea there is no obstruction in the throat. Rather it's an uncommon problem of the brain not properly controlling the breathing when asleep. It does occur in normal people, however, particularly as they get older. Obesity is usually not a factor.

One clue that might mean you have central sleep apnea is whether you sometimes awaken during the night with a feeling you are choking. You may even run to the window to get air. This behavior is common in central sleep apnea but uncommon in the obstructive variety.

Keep in mind, however, that sleep apneas of both sorts can be dangerous if they decrease the amount of oxygen in the blood or make the heart beat too fast, too slowly, or irregularly. These factors can lead to heart disease and are a major cause of death during sleep.

The treatment of central sleep apnea is not pleasant. If you have a severe case, it may require mechanical ventilation by a respirator. One bright spot is that if central sleep apnea is caused by congestive heart failure (the heart does not pump strongly enough and thus the lungs fill with fluid) it can be eliminated by medical therapy. Congestive heart failure is a far more common medical problem than most people realize.

An obstruction in the nose can also cause central sleep apnea. The obstruction lowers the level of oxygen in the blood, which in turn results in less oxygen being delivered to the brain, affecting the brain's control of breathing during sleep. Except for the usual colds and other illnesses that affect the nose, no one really understands why a healthy nose may become obstructed. There are nerves in the nose that regulate respiration but it is not clear why the nose should "close up" in some people.

**INSURANCE REIMBURSEMENT** A big problem with disorders of excessive sleepiness is insurance coverage. While sleep apnea is well recognized today and most insurance companies will pay for diagnosis and treatment, other sleep disorders are not. Therefore many doctors who may feel the patient has, for example, excessive daytime sleepiness, cause as yet undetermined, will instead write down *sleep apnea*.

Some doctors, in fact, automatically write *sleep apnea* as a diagnosis for everyone with any kind of sleep disorder. This white lie poses a possible problem for the patient. *Sleep apnea* will appear in the records of your insurance company. Since sleep apnea is a serious, potentially fatal disease, the diagnosis may get in the way of your ability to get health and life insurance in the future. Doctors have been sued by irate patients for just this reason.

These considerations are much more pressing if your health insurance is handled by an HMO, where the doctor is paid a fixed amount per month to take care of all health care no matter what is wrong with you. Testing for sleep disorders by polysomnography lasts all night and often must be done on successive nights because the patient does not feel comfortable initially and will not sleep well. As a result, it is expensive. And HMOs, as a matter of cost containment, may give both subtle and direct hints to their doctors to do as little as possible. If you believe that you have sleep apnea, ask your physician to order polysomnography. If he refuses, ask why. If you are not satisfied, ask about an appeal procedure.

## ABNORMAL SLEEP BEHAVIOR (PARASOMNIA)

Finally we come to some of the stranger sleep disorders, the parasomnias. These are abnormal behaviors that, although they may seem funny to some, particularly those that involve thrashing, they can be a real problem if you have them or have to live with someone who does.

One difficulty you may encounter with regard to parasomnias is that many doctors are unaware of some of them. It's not that these behaviors are often confused with something else or that your doctor might offer an inappropriate treatment, it's that he or she may simply treat you like a child with a fantasy when you speak of them.

**DISORDERS OF EXCESSIVE SLEEPINESS** I've already touched on this problem as symptomatic of other sleep disorders, but here I deal with it as a separate insomnia. I first experienced it myself when I was an intern. Today I see it when a patient comes in complaining of just feeling sleepy all the time. As I've indicated earlier, the desired treatment is removing the cause. But sometimes that can't be done (or there is no apparent cause), so it simply must be treated by itself.

This was the case with one seventeen-year-old I saw recently. He was failing in school because he was always nodding off and could not stay awake long enough to do his homework.

Many sleepy patients have come to see me since I became known as a specialist in Chronic Fatigue Syndrome (CFS) and since sleep disorders are an important part of this disease (see Chapter 4). This boy did not become fatigued and had no problems with exercise, as he would have with CFS. Obviously he did not have CFS; he was just sleepy most of the time.

His family doctor had done the usual tests, all of which were negative. The boy had then been sent to a psychiatrist and had been treated for depression, of which he had no other symptoms at all. Sleepiness can indeed be a symptom of depression, but depression is characterized by an early onset of REM sleep at night and an increased amount of REM during the total sleep period. Although most depressives sleep less than normal and experience early-morning awakening, a subgroup of depressed patients sleep more than normal. He did not fit this mold.

This boy did not snore and was not fat, but he recalled a few short periods of amnesia when he did things he did not remember, such as driving on the freeway and ending up someplace he had never been before or putting his books in the refrigerator. These spells are called automatic behavior and are also seen in other sleep disorders.

I referred him for sleep monitoring, the results of which were normal. I then assumed that he had narcolepsy, but he was not positive for the common narcoleptic genetic marker HLA-DR2, and repeated testing did not show the immediate REM-sleep phenomenon also found in narcolepsy.

We were left with the diagnosis of a sleep disorder of unknown cause. He had had mononucleosis several months before this behavior started, and the two events could have been related. A virus could have caused a malfunction of the areas of the brain that maintain wakefulness. Treatment involved long-term drug therapy directly intended to help him maintain wakefulness during the day.

This disorder can be mild; you may simply nod off while watching TV or reading. Or it can be more severe, like getting very sleepy while driving. One executive who was having a dinner party for his senior management knew it was important for future career advancement, and he and his wife had spent days making sure everything was just right. The mood was definitely spoiled when, right in the middle of the main course, he fell asleep facedown in his mashed potatoes.

**SLEEPWALKING AND NIGHT TERRORS**  Sleepwalking is relatively more common in children than in adults. It usually requires a physician's care if it occurs so often that the child may hurt himself or seriously disturb the family.

Night terrors are also fairly common, usually in children,

when screaming and fearful, sometimes violent behavior occurs. When this happens more than rarely, professional attention is called for. Occasionally sleepwalking and night terrors occur together.

It is important that, when you do see your physician, he or she doesn't give your child a pat on the head and say, "He will outgrow it." Indeed this might happen. But it also might not. Sleepwalking and night terrors may actually be a variation of a seizure disorder, since the victim may be confused afterward and lack a clear memory of what happened.

A physician should check to be sure there are no other physical or emotional problems involved and should also be concerned that the patient doesn't hurt himself or herself during the episodes. Sleepwalking and night terrors may be physical manifestations of psychological trauma or conflict.

If brain abnormalities are seen in testing, it is worth trying medication that decreases spontaneous electrical activity in the temporal regions. Your doctor may want to try drugs such as carbamazepine (Tegretol), valproic acid (Depakote), and/or clonazepam (Klonopin), which has the added advantage of suppressing both REM and NREM sleep. These do not always work, however. When they don't, counseling may provide some help.

**THRASHING OR ARM AND LEG MOVEMENT**  Sometimes a person actually tries to act out a dream, particularly when it is very vivid, frightening, or violent. Of course, since normally when we dream we are in REM sleep and paralysis is a condition of REM, this is not usually possible. However, sometimes things don't work that way.

Sometimes a person does not have the usual muscle inhibition that occurs during REM sleep. A common story is that one spouse attacks another in the middle of the night imagining he or she is behaving in a threatening or assaultive manner. Running or other evasive or thrashing kinds of behavior and talking or yelling during sleep is frequently found in this disorder.

This problem is technically termed a REM sleep behavior disorder, since the paralysis of normal REM sleep somehow does not function. It can be caused by various drugs, drug withdrawal, or illnesses, often viral. These kinds of behaviors are reported rather frequently when I take histories of Chronic Fatigue Syndrome patients.

Again, your doctor may first jump to the conclusion that a marital or psychological problem exists and immediately suggest psychiatric treatment.

While that may be necessary eventually, it is always best to first try to see if the problem isn't organic. Therefore it is very important that the physician do tests to make sure the behavior is occurring during REM sleep and also to demonstrate that it is not a seizure. I do not believe a diagnosis of partial complex seizures can always be made with certainty by the conventional paper electroencephalogram (EEG) which records brain waves. A BEAM scan* is a more appropriate diagnostic tool.

For a REM-sleep behavior disorder, your doctor may want to use Klonopin, which reduces seizures and anxiety and is very effective in REM-sleep behavior disorder, usually at a fairly low dosage. It should go without saying that if you have any of the problems described above, you should also have a bedroom that minimizes the chances of injury.

## RESTLESS LEGS SYNDROME AND PERIODIC MOVEMENTS DURING SLEEP    These are two other fairly common parasomnias.

The restless leg syndrome usually occurs in the evening, especially at bedtime, and consists of a "creepy-crawly" sensation associated with an inability to keep your legs still. These problems occur in both legs simultaneously and are not caused by other nervous-system diseases.

These disorders are not serious, but may delay your falling asleep and occasionally spread to other parts of the body. They have always reminded me of a disorder called akathisia, in which the patient has an inability to keep his or her legs still and constantly feels the need to walk. Medications that stop akathisia, however, may have little value if you have restless leg syndrome. Only the drug L-dopa, which is converted to dopamine, has been systematically evaluated and been found to be effective.

If you have restless leg syndrome, you may have excessive

---

*A BEAM scan is Brain Electrical Activity Mapping, a new technique which uses computer analysis to compare brain activity in a patient to a large group of normal people.

daytime sleepiness as well. The disorder may come and go in a manner that is difficult to explain. It is probably hereditary.

Adding to the peculiarity of this disorder is the fact that once a person with restless leg syndrome falls asleep, the big toe as well as the entire foot usually flex up (dorsiflexion), often accompanied by flexing of the knee and hip. These bizarre movements last about a second and may occur every twenty to forty seconds. If severe, they can frequently awaken you. You may feel like you've just run a marathon every morning, and, in actuality, you may have come close to doing just that. This disorder occurs mainly in non-REM sleep, when muscle movement is not inhibited.

I have found that the drug Klonopin has been most frequently reported to be effective. It may act by decreasing NREM sleep or by reducing the excitability of certain nerves. Opioid (opium-related) drugs are also quite effective, and many patients take propoxyphene (Darvon) at bedtime with little addiction liability at a low dose. An L-dopa/carbidopa (Sinemet) combination is also effective and may work better in the elderly. L-dopa may also make your sleep less fragmented, something that normally occurs in the elderly. It also, surprisingly, may help with narcolepsy.

**TOOTH-GRINDING**  This disorder, called bruxism, may also involve jaw-clenching during sleep, is a very common condition, and is apparently hereditary. I consider it the most common cause of headache upon awakening.

It can be particularly painful; the jaw and temple muscles are almost always tender in bruxers. It can also be an aspect of fibromyalgia (see Chapter 1) and can occur in both REM and non-REM sleep, although some believe the REM variety more destructive. Bruxism can be severe in times of personal stress.

The major problem here is that the pain or headache occurs when the patient is awake and the doctor may confuse the disorder with any number of other problems, from migraine to jaw-joint problems (temporomandibular pain). Usually a clear indication is a wearing away of the teeth, so that dentists are often the first to come up with an accurate diagnosis. It should be ruled out before looking elsewhere for the cause of your headache.

The first step in treating this problem is to determine at what stage in sleep the grinding or clenching occurs. Your doctor may want to use tricyclic antidepressants if the bruxism occurs during REM sleep (they suppress REM) and Klonopin if most of the bruxism takes place during REM or NREM sleep. On numerous occasions I have had a patient with intractable head and face pain and resistant to other measures joyfully exclaim something like ''My jaw just popped open'' when the proper dose of Klonopin was reached. Your dentist can also make a plastic splint for you to wear at night that may decrease your symptoms.

## TO LEARN MORE

There are by now many sources for information on sleep disorders: a society of subspecialists in sleep medicine involving neurology, psychiatry, cardiology, and pulmonology for the most part, a journal devoted entirely to the topic (appropriately entitled *Sleep*), and several recent books. The one I have found most valuable and comprehensive and fairly readable for the layperson is *Principles and Practice of Sleep Medicine,* edited by Meir H. Kryger, Thomas Roth, and William C. Dement (Philadelphia: W. B. Saunders, 1989).

# 3

=

# Senility/Dementia

*Senility* is what we used to call a condition in the elderly when they had a lot of trouble remembering and handling such tasks as driving a car that they had previously done with ease. Over time the term *senile* itself began to be applied disparagingly to any elderly person having problems thinking. For the remainder of this chapter I will therefore use *dementia*, a term that is not as emotionally loaded and is more technically accurate.

Dementia is not limited to old people: It can happen at any age. In fact, age itself is not the cause, but rather it comes about from a variety of disease processes. If you or a friend or relative suffers from apparent dementia, read this chapter very carefully. You may find diagnoses and treatments in this chapter which are quite different from those you have already received.

## WHAT IS DEMENTIA?

According to the psychiatrist's bible, the *Diagnostic and Statistical Manual* (DSM-III-R), ''The essential feature of dementia is impairment in short- and long-term memory, associated with impairment in abstract thinking, impaired judgement, other disturbances of higher control function, or personality change. The disturbance is severe enough to interfere significantly with work or usual social activities or relationships with others.''

Most physicians associate dementia with Alzheimer's disease. This disorder can begin slowly but can become completely disabling. Of course, dementia can have other causes and be confused with other conditions, including:

AIDS
Alcohol abuse
Brain injury
Brain tumor
Chemical intoxication of various kinds
Chronic Fatigue Syndrome
Drug abuse, particularly of cocaine
Hormonal problems
Huntington disease
Inflammation
Kidney failure
Liver failure
Multiple brain-artery blockages
Multiple sclerosis
Parkinson disease
Vitamin $B_{12}$ deficiency

Other generalized diseases can affect brain function, including pseudodementia.

**FALSE DEMENTIA (PSEUDODEMENTIA)**   Sometimes a diagnosis of dementia or impairment of brain function is inaccurate. Yes, your elderly mother does have trouble remembering; you can see she's slowing down, not moving as fast as she used to. She doesn't care about anything. But does this automatically mean that she has dementia?

Not necessarily. She could have false dementia brought on by depression. It's very important for your doctor to find out which it is, because pseudodementia is treatable with antidepressants, whereas true dementia is not.

Since it is sometimes hard to tell which is which, discuss with your doctor trying antidepressant therapy. If pseudodementia is present, the cognitive problems will largely disappear and the patient will feel a great deal more cheerful. On the other hand, if there is no improvement, the condition is probably true dementia. (Sometimes depression occurs as a part of the Alzheimer's type of dementia. In this case antidepressants may significantly improve intellectual functions, although obviously there will not be any recovery of dead nerve cells.)

Another way pseudodementia may be diagnosed is by a SPECT scan, a computerized technique to measure brain blood flow.* People with pseudodementia will not have reductions in blood flow in the characteristic areas for Alzheimer's disease.

Pseudodementia is fairly common. The aware physician has the opportunity to greatly alter a person's quality of life by ordering an antidepressant.

## DEMENTIA IN AIDS

A problem that is less frequently dealt with appropriately is dementia in people with AIDS. Sometimes in the initial stages of AIDS, the only abnormalities may be alteration of brain function, which may be quite severe. These people are often misdiagnosed as having severe depression or schizophrenia and some have been placed in psychiatric wards.

There are possible new treatments for this problem, technically called AIDS encephalopathy. One ingenious experiment has found that certain cells (macrophages) in the brains of AIDS patients may secrete toxic substances. It may be possible to block this process.

## DEMENTIA IN CHRONIC FATIGUE SYNDROME

The most common dementia I see in my practice is related to Chronic Fatigue Syndrome (CFS), in which it is a very common symptom that produces one of the truly great areas of misdiagnosis occurring today. Many doctors still think that Chronic Fatigue Syndrome is only a form of depression and, consequently, end up prescribing antidepressants. The real problem, of course, Chronic Fatigue Syndrome, remains undiagnosed and unaddressed.

**DISTINGUISHING CFS DEMENTIA FROM DEPRESSION** For the doctor who understands that CFS does exist and knows the symptoms, it is quite easy to distinguish between dementia brought on by the illness and that brought on by depression. For example, in psychological testing, depressed people have slowed responses but are still accurate. CFS patients have problems with information processing of various sorts, particu-

*SPECT scans use computer analysis of radioactive gas that is inhaled and a substance that is intravenously injected to measure how much radioactivity travels through the blood vessels of the brain.

larly the encoding of new memories. Consequently they are both slow and inaccurate. Further, dementia in CFS can be profound, rendering people unable to read, drive, work, balance checkbooks, remember their children's names, or what to do when a traffic light changes. This deficit is more severe than would normally be encountered with depression.

Other ways to differentiate between dementia caused by Chronic Fatigue Syndrome and depression include the presence of other disorders and symptoms typically seen as part of the CFS spectrum. These include fibromyalgia, irritable bowel syndrome, allergic rhinitis, and premenstrual syndrome. All of these may have elements of dementia associated with them. Once the cause is treated, the mild dementia associated with these separate disorders often responds as well.

## SPECIAL DEMENTIA DIAGNOSTIC TECHNIQUES

If there is possibility of a dementia disorder, you need the help of a physician. You really can't find out yourself.

Ask your physician about certain tests. Some of these involve sophisticated computerized tests such as BEAM, SPECT, or PET scans and are often expensive. Even so, they are invaluable for a conclusive diagnosis.*

## USING DRUGS TO TREAT DEMENTIA

You should talk with your physician about the use of certain drugs that may help certain dementias. In particular you may

---

*My understanding of dementias, particularly in younger people, has been greatly enhanced by the use of "functional brain imaging," a process which measures electrical, blood flow, metabolic and electromagnetic activity in the brain rather than taking a picture of it as MRI and CT scans do. The brain may look normal but not function properly. These sorts of tests are not well known by most physicians, and their potential remains largely untapped.

Recently, a technique called "evoked responses," or "evoked potentials" has been developed in which a visual, auditory or bodily stimulus is given and the electrical message is plotted as it travels through the brain. Computer analysis of the EEG and evoked response data has resulted in what is called "topographic brain mapping," in which the computer generates a colored picture of the varying intensities of electrical activity gathered by EEG and evoked response measurement. In the best systems (as far as I am concerned), the electrical data is analyzed by the computer and then compared to a large number of normal people who had brain mapping done under very strict criteria. The maps of the brain then tell the neurologist how different from normal are the results he is seeing.

want to ask about Hydergine. Hydergine is used mainly in the United States for senile dementia Alzheimer type (SDAT), which it helps slightly. It may help dementias in younger people more profoundly, but must usually be given in higher doses than are recommended by the manufacturer. A drug that is used to treat blood flow problems, nimodipine (Nimotop), shows promise in treating SDAT as well as dementias in younger people.

## OTHER TREATMENTS

Choline and lecithin, which can be purchased as nutritional supplements, help some patients to think better. Piracetam also produced a mild improvement in dyslexia in a large study. This drug may work for dementia as well, but I am not convinced the results are real and not enhanced by the expectations of those taking it. You may want to discuss this medication with your physician. It is available in many other countries, but not in the United States. Drugs related to piracetam, such as aniracetam, may be more effective.

---

I have done BEAM scans on young patients with dementias related to CFS and they are usually abnormal, most frequently in the temporal lobes. Sometimes these patients will respond to temporal lobe medications such as carbamazepine (Tegretol), valproic acid (Depakote) or clonazepam (Klonopin). When their general illness gets better and their thinking improves the BEAM scan will also become more normal.

SPECT (Single Photon Emission Computerized Tomography) scans show regional blood flow in the brain. Originally used in strokes, SPECT scans are having a wider and wider applicability, since many brain disorders apparently have variations in blood flow, usually decreases. Sometimes the blood flow can be increased by drugs.

PET (Positron Emission Tomography) scans measure metabolism of sugar in the brain. Areas of the brain that are not working properly do not use as much sugar.

BEAM, SPECT and PET scans can be done "dynamically," as the patient does different tasks to activate different regions of the brain, and radioactive drugs can be used in SPECT and PET scans to label receptors for brain chemicals to further define what might be wrong in "neurotransmitters," and could lead to more intelligent treatment of many disorders. This technology is available right now, but is underutilized because of lack of physician awareness, lack of research funding, and (particularly) poor insurance reimbursement for these procedures.

# 4

# Chronic Fatigue Syndrome

"I had the flu and it just never seemed to clear up. I lay in bed and used to worry if I would have the energy to get up and get to the bathroom. It went on for months and months."

Karen was describing her case of Chronic Fatigue Syndrome (CFS). This debilitating illness affects thousands, perhaps millions, of Americans. It is a disorder that is of great interest to the general public. It is also frequently confused with several other illnesses, including depression, which we will discuss in Chapter 13. Over the past few years, more out of necessity than design, I have become a specialist in this illness, as thousands of patients who could not get help elsewhere have besieged me. In this chapter I want both to describe the strange and newly recognized disease and impart an understanding of where we are in fighting it.

Of course, Karen went to her doctor—during the following two years she went to over a dozen doctors. At various times she was diagnosed as having Lyme disease, multiple sclerosis, hyperthyroidism, hepatitis, and lymphoma (a cancer). Finally she was told she had acute depression and that she should seek the services of a psychiatrist. In other words, the disease was all in her mind. Still believing in her doctors, she went.

Fortunately, the psychiatrist she went to had heard of her illness and correctly diagnosed it as Chronic Fatigue and Immune Dysfunction Syndrome, usually known as Chronic Fatigue Syndrome (CFS). Her doctor was able to put her in touch with a physician who knew how to treat the illness and today she is better.

What's unfortunate is that Karen's case is not unusual. A vast majority of Chronic Fatigue Syndrome sufferers experience similar fates. They contract an illness that completely

**61**

wipes them out and then, when they go to their physicians for treatment, they are either misdiagnosed or referred to some other specialist. It is not uncommon for a patient in these circumstances to ping-pong from doctor to doctor, usually at a cost of tens of thousands of dollars in often inappropriate diagnostic tests, all for nothing, since the patient is not helped by these medical efforts.

## THE ROLE OF THE MEDICAL ESTABLISHMENT

Chronic Fatigue Syndrome is the perfect example of the problems today's patient faces. Chronic Fatigue Syndrome is a new disease, at least in the minds of doctors. (It may actually have been around for a great many years.) It may cause its symptoms in a novel manner, and doesn't fit the way medical science understands things. In short, it isn't listed in the medical cookbook most doctors use. Hence they feel at a loss when it comes to dealing with it.

The medical establishment has badly mishandled the Chronic Fatigue Syndrome problem. There is great reluctance on the part of physicians to think that the way medical science looks at things may be the culprit. A great many patients have been left to suffer needlessly.

## THE SEARCH FOR CHRONIC FATIGUE SYNDROME

Chronic Fatigue Syndrome may have been with us for several centuries. However, it did not receive much attention until a series of recent "epidemics" broke out and brought it notoriety.

The best-documented of these happened in the Lake Tahoe area around Incline Village in late 1984. At that time doctors began to see a large number of patients with flulike symptoms. What was unusual was that they all seemed to have incapacitating fatigue and weakness that did not respond to antibiotics and did not clear up, month after month.

This syndrome at first produced derision. It was called the Yuppie Flu, since most of the patients were young urban professionals. It also was dubbed the Raggedy Ann syndrome since the patients were so without energy that they tended to come in looking like rag dolls.

However, as a tide of cases came into doctors' offices, it soon became apparent that what was appearing was a new kind of illness (new to doctors). A number of dedicated physicians began to attempt to understand this illness and were rewarded for their efforts often by being derided and having their findings ignored by other physicians.

Dr. Anthony L. Komaroff, associate professor of medicine at Harvard and chief of general medicine at Brigham and Women's Hospital in Boston, thinks that Chronic Fatigue Syndrome may be caused by activation of dormant viruses and other infectious agents which cause some people's immune systems to act in an inappropriate way to cause this disease.

The search for Chronic Fatigue Syndrome has also been hampered by the fact that those seriously involved in research have themselves not been able to come up with a definitive diagnosis. I make the diagnosis by excluding other illnesses that may have similar characteristics and performing tests that will indicate activation of the immune system and characteristic dysfunction of the brain.

## RELATIONSHIP TO THE EPSTEIN–BARR VIRUS

One of the first discoveries was that a large number of patients with Chronic Fatigue Syndrome also had Epstein–Barr virus.* Doctors jumped the gun and added two and two together only to get five; many made the assumption that since Epstein–Barr virus antibodies were present, the virus must be causing this disease. In 1985 and 1986 a great deal of notoriety was given to the Epstein–Barr virus, with physicians writing books on the subject and appearing as guests on television talks shows to discuss this idea.

Unfortunately, they were premature. What we've discovered is that although Epstein–Barr may play a role in this disease, it is not the causative agent.

When this finding became generally known and accepted, it tended to make those physicians who had gone public about Epstein–Barr look a bit foolish. It also tended to cast doubt on the validity of the illness in the minds of the public. To many

---

*Epstein–Barr virus is one of the six herpes viruses. It causes infectious mononucleosis and a cancer of the nose and throat. Otherwise, the virus has not been related to illnesses frequently encountered in the United States.

on the sidelines who only know what they read in the news-
papers or see on TV, it appeared that their physicians and
researchers were indeed charlatans.

When the assertion that the illness was due to the Epstein–
Barr virus was discredited (or so it appeared), the disorder was
renamed Chronic Fatigue Syndrome. To this day patients ask
"Do I have Chronic Fatigue Syndrome or Epstein–Barr?"

This confusion is most unfortunate, since we are talking
about a very serious—though not usually fatal—disorder that
afflicts a great many people. The illness does exist, and if you
have it, you should not have to bear the brunt of skepticism
from those who think you must have a mental problem.

Current research into the cause of Chronic Fatigue Syndrome
has centered on what has been termed Agent X. Agent X may be
a virus that, perhaps in conjunction with a toxic agent, produces a
deficiency in the immune systems of certain genetically susceptible people. Once the change in the immune system occurs, it allows the patient to become susceptible to other viruses, such as
the human herpes virus 6 (HHV-6), as well as to other sorts of
stressors that could activate the disease.

## WHO GETS CHRONIC FATIGUE SYNDROME?

Today we realize that many people can develop Chronic
Fatigue Syndrome. Adults under the age of forty-five seem
most susceptible, and a majority of patients are women.

Chronic Fatigue Syndrome is a psychoneuroimmunologic
disorder. This means that it has elements of psychological,
neurological, and immunological dysfunction. As mentioned,
it appears that a genetic predisposition toward the illness may
be a factor. Prior illness, environment, and stress as well as
age and gender may also be factors. Patients with CFS have
an immune system that is continually activated without an obvious reason. The immune activation and accompanying brain
dysfunction produce the characteristic symptoms.

## HOW MANY PEOPLE HAVE
## CHRONIC FATIGUE SYNDROME?

It's not really possible to say, since no accurate statistical
studies have so far been done. I have seen over two thou-

sand CFS patients in the past five years. As word has gotten out that this is indeed a treatable illness, my patient load has increased geometrically until it is almost overwhelming. This same phenomenon has been reported by other physicians across the country (and, indeed, around the world) who are also researching the syndrome and treating Chronic Fatigue Syndrome patients. I have heard others say that there are two million to six million people in the United States alone who have the disease, but I really don't trust those figures. A recent study in Germany has suggested that the actual rate of infection may be four out of a thousand, but I am not sure how this rate was determined, either. Research being done by Australian physicians and by the Centers for Disease Control in four American cities should help us make a more precise estimate.

## DIAGNOSING CHRONIC FATIGUE SYNDROME

First of all it's important to understand what Chronic Fatigue Syndrome is *not*. It is not simple chronic fatigue. You may feel tired all the time, but that does not necessarily mean that you have Chronic Fatigue Syndrome. The symptoms of Chronic Fatigue Syndrome include much more than simple fatigue. Simply being tired may mean that you are anemic or that you have some other problem that is relatively easy to diagnose and treat.

Chronic Fatigue Syndrome is not depression. Chronic Fatigue Syndrome patients are often depressed, but that is a symptom of the illness, not the cause. Too often unthinking physicians have dropped Chronic Fatigue Syndrome patients into the medical wastebasket called depression. Since they couldn't find an appropriate answer, they resorted to the old dodge "It's all in the mind." Of course, they forget that the mind is indeed connected to the body. Depression is a distinct problem, and those suffering from depression typically do not have many of such other characteristic symptoms of Chronic Fatigue Syndrome as a sore throat.

What, then, is Chronic Fatigue Syndrome? The answer is not easy to give, since the symptoms are variable and there is no well accepted laboratory test to diagnose the disease and determine its severity. Doctors must rule out every other possible disease before they can say you have CFS. To understand this situation, consider chickenpox. When a person has chickenpox, there are definite and dramatic signs that anybody, not merely a physician, can see. Besides the fever, there is the pox itself. I can't imagine two physicians arguing over whether or not someone has typical chickenpox.

Unfortunately, Chronic Fatigue Syndrome is quite the opposite. Usually the symptoms are quite numerous, they may wax and wane, and they can be symptomatic of many other diseases. In addition, the symptoms do not fall within a single medical discipline but instead cross many boundaries. (They overlap the areas of general medicine, rheumatology, allergy, infectious diseases, psychiatry, neurology, and immunology.) Thus no one discipline has been willing to embrace the disease.

As a result, there has been a stubborn reluctance in the medical community even to admit that Chronic Fatigue Syndrome exists, let alone to treat it. However, since the Centers for Disease Control in Atlanta officially acknowledged this illness, the reluctance has begun to fade.

In the March 1988 issue of *Annals of Internal Medicine*, Dr. Gary Holmes of the Centers for Disease Control (CDC) along with 15 other physicians, published an article in which they presented a "working case definition" for the illness. The most significant aspect of this definition is that it gave an official stamp to the disease and helped legitimize it.

However, it must be understood that the working case definition presented was based on the best information obtainable at the time and that research since then has moved forward quickly and dramatically.


## SYMPTOM CHECKLIST

Do you have Chronic Fatigue Syndrome? I encourage you to go through the following checklist. It lists the symptoms other researchers and I have found for Chronic Fatigue Syndrome and gives the approximate percentages of CFS patients who suffer from the symptoms. Rate the severity of your symptoms from 0 to 10. Remember that this checklist is not diagnostic, but a high percentage of items checked is indicative of the possibility of having CFS.

1. \_\_Fatigue (95%)—usually made worse by exercise
2. \_\_Cognitive function problems (80%)
   \_\_a. attention deficit disorder
   \_\_b. calculation difficulties
   \_\_c. memory disturbance
   \_\_d. spatial disorientation
   \_\_e. frequently saying the wrong word
3. \_\_Psychological problems (80%)
   \_\_a. depression
   \_\_b. anxiety—which may include panic attacks
   \_\_c. personality changes—usually a worsening of a previous mild tendency
   \_\_d. emotional lability (mood swings)
   \_\_e. psychosis (1%)
4. \_\_Other nervous system problems (75%)
   \_\_a. sleep disturbance
   \_\_b. headaches
   \_\_c. changes in visual acuity
   \_\_d. seizures
   \_\_e. numb or tingling feelings
   \_\_f. vertigo
   \_\_g. lightheadedness—feeling "spaced-out"
   \_\_h. frequent unusual nightmares
   \_\_i. difficulty moving tongue to speak
   \_\_j. ringing in ears
   \_\_k. paralysis
   \_\_l. severe muscular weakness
   \_\_m. blackouts
   \_\_n. intolerance of bright lights
   \_\_o. intolerance of alcohol
   \_\_p. alteration of taste, smell, hearing
   \_\_q. nonrestorative sleep
   \_\_r. decreased libido (sex drive)
   \_\_s. twitching muscles ("benign fasciculations")
5. \_\_Recurrent flulike illnesses (75%)—often with chronic sore throat
6. \_\_Painful lymph nodes—especially on sides of neck and under the arms (60%)
7. \_\_Severe nasal and other allergies—often worsening of previous mild problem (40%)
8. \_\_Weight change—usually gain (70%)

9. \_\_Muscle and joint aches with tender ''trigger points'' or fibromyalgia (65%)
10. \_\_Abdominal pain, diarrhea, nausea, intestinal gas—irritable bowel syndrome (50%)
11. \_\_Low-grade fevers or feeling hot often (70%)
12. \_\_Night sweats (40%)
13. \_\_Heart palpitations (40%)
14. \_\_Severe premenstrual syndrome—PMS (70% of women)
15. \_\_Rash of herpes simplex or shingles (20%)
16. \_\_Uncomfortable or recurrent urination—pain in prostate (20%)
17. \_\_Other symptoms seen in varying percentages of patients
    \_\_a. rashes
    \_\_b. hair loss
    \_\_c. impotence
    \_\_d. chest pain
    \_\_e. dry eyes and mouth
    \_\_f. cough
    \_\_g. TMJ syndrome
    \_\_h. mitral valve prolapse
    \_\_i. frequent canker sores
    \_\_j. cold hands and feet
    \_\_k. serious rhythm disturbances of the heart
    \_\_l. carpal tunnel syndrome
    \_\_m. pyriform muscle syndrome causing sciatica
    \_\_n. thyroid inflammation
    \_\_o. various cancers (a rare occurrence)
    \_\_p. periodontal (gum) disease
    \_\_q. endometriosis
    \_\_r. easily getting out of breath (''dyspnea on exertion'')
    \_\_s. Symptoms worsened by extremes of temperature
    \_\_t. Multiple sensitivities to medicines, food, and other substances

(Note: Some of the above statistics were compiled with the assistance of data provided by several researchers in this field.)

## DRAMATIC SYMPTOMS

Perhaps the most debilitating feature of Chronic Fatigue Syndrome besides the fatigue is the way it can transform a functional human being into someone operating on an almost vegetative level. I have seen IQ scores drop thirty points for victims of Chronic Fatigue Syndrome. I have a doctor as a patient who can no longer drive a car because he can't read the street signs. He doesn't understand what it means when the light is green, yellow, or red. I have mothers who can't remember the names of their sons and daughters.

This loss usually corresponds to what is seen in certain scans of the brain's functional activity (since the brain and the immune system can almost be thought of as one organ) that show there are characteristic brain lesions in most of the people who have Chronic Fatigue Syndrome.

## CONFUSION WITH OTHER ILLNESS

It is important to understand that, just like chickenpox or polio or AIDS, Chronic Fatigue Syndrome is a definable disease. However, because it is complex and difficult to diagnose, understand, and deal with, it is sometimes confused with other illnesses. At this point there is no one test that will definitely diagnose CFS. The following is a list of other syndromes that are sometimes confused with Chronic Fatigue Syndrome. You may want to discuss this list with your physician if you have been diagnosed as having one of these illnesses yet have the symptoms of Chronic Fatigue Syndrome, or if you have been diagnosed as having CFS but are getting worse.

1. Toxoplasmosis (an infection with a microorganism called a protozoan which causes enlarged lymph nodes, among its other symptoms)
2. Collagen vascular disease, especially lupus
3. Lyme arthritis (Lyme disease)
4. AIDS or AIDS-related complex
5. Multiple sclerosis
6. Anxiety disorders
7. Psychophysiologic disorders

8. Mucocutaneous candidiasis (a yeast infection)
9. Hypothyroidism
10. Immune deficiency states
11. Parasitic infection (Giardia)
12. Chronic active hepatitis
13. Cancer (especially lymphoma)
14. Tuberculosis
15. Brucellosis (a bacterial infection that causes relapsing fatigue and fever, sometimes contracted from drinking unpasteurized milk)
16. Anemia
17. Multiple drug use/drug effects/drug interactions
18. Subacute bacterial endocarditis (a bacterial infection of the heart valves that can spread clumps of bacteria throughout the body via the bloodstream)
19. Sleep disorders
20. Depression
21. Somatization disorder (a conversion of psychological conflicts into multiple physical symptoms)

## WHAT HAPPENS TO
## CHRONIC FATIGUE SYNDROME PATIENTS?

Almost no one dies of Chronic Fatigue Syndrome, but the malady is long-lived. Those who do not seek treatment are typically debilitated for a very long period of time, months to (often) years. Of those who do seek treatment and reach a doctor who understands their problem, about 80 percent can be helped. This means we can get these people back to leading productive lives. It does not mean that if you have CFS we can cure you or alleviate all symptoms of the disease. As of now, we do not fully understand the illness, nor do we have a cure for it.

## WHAT CAN YOU DO IF YOU HAVE
## CHRONIC FATIGUE SYNDROME?

This illness can be very frustrating. As suggested by Karen's case, as well as by my experiences with hundreds of other patients, dealing with this illness is difficult.

For one thing, it's important to understand that you need

help. Regardless of what some early so-called authorities have said in print and on television, you are *unlikely* to be helped by simply taking nutritional supplements or by exercising. Exercise, in fact, usually makes the disease worse, which may distinguish it from fibromyalgia (see Chapter 1).

Cases of spontaneous remission, where the illness suddenly disappears as mysteriously as it came, are the exception. In most cases, if you do nothing you will find that you are incapacitated for a very long time. This can be psychologically draining, financially ruinous, and has led to the breakup of families.

On the other hand, if you go to your family practitioner and he is not well versed in CFS, you may only be adding to your woes. There is amazing inertia among physicians, even this late in the game, when it comes to dealing with Chronic Fatigue Syndrome.

Typically, the physician prescribes a standard battery of tests for a wide variety of illnesses that must be ruled out before Chronic Fatigue Syndrome can be diagnosed with certainty. Naturally enough, when the test results come back negative (since they were tests for other illnesses) the doctor will be frustrated. The illness doesn't fit his cookbook recipe. He may tell you nothing can be done for you and that you should just go home and rest. He may prescribe an antidepressant. (This can actually help sometimes, but will certainly not cure the problem.)

Or he may fasten on one or more symptoms and refer you to a specialist. The specialist will again perform a battery of tests for illnesses with which he is familiar. When these come back negative (again because they were for other illnesses), he too may be frustrated and refer you on to yet another specialist. You end up on a round of doctor-hopping and taking test after test. Besides the enormous financial burden there is a drain on the patient's emotional resources.

In case after case this process has taken place or the physician simply does not take the patient seriously. The most common diagnosis targets psychological problems—doctors focus on the patient's depression. Since Chronic Fatigue Syndrome patients tend to be depressed anyway (as a symptom of the illness, not a cause), it is easier for many physicians to explain the illness away on these grounds than to accept the challenge of dealing with it. In defense of these doctors, most have little time to spend with you, are overworked, or belong to health maintenance organizations where the emphasis may be on low-cost, simplistic, or palliative solutions.

## WHAT SHOULD YOU DO?

What you must do if you have the illness is find an enlightened physician who can help you deal with it. There are more and more such physicians across the country as this disease gains credibility. (You can find these through the Chronic Fatigue and Immune Dysfunction Syndrome Association, telephone 704-362-CFID.) Newsletters that publish the latest information on the disease can also be a source of physicians. The largest of these is the *CFIDS Chronicle*, (Box 220398, Charlotte, NC 28222-0398), which has some 20,000 subscribers.

In addition, Chronic Fatigue Syndrome support groups have sprung up around the country. These organizations provide psychological support and encouragement as well as usually accurate advice on how to get medical, legal, and financial aid.

And you should take another look at the symptom checklist. This will help you to determine in your own mind if you have this illness.

## UNDERSTANDING AND TREATING CFS

To help my patients understand Chronic Fatigue Syndrome I have developed an approach for treating the illness that I believe helps to conceptualize it. This approach may also help you understand the complexity of CFS.

I regard Chronic Fatigue Syndrome as a "psychoneuroimmunologic" disorder. That means that it has aspects of at least three separate disciplines:

1. Psychology—affecting the thinking and emotions of the patient.
2. Neurology—affecting the brain itself in a chemical way.
3. Immunology—affecting the body's immune system.

My method is to break the disease down into six separate phases, from phase zero to phase five. Each phase is a different way in which the illness manifests itself to the observer. While there is a tendency to see the disease as a progression from phase zero to phase five, in actuality the phases usually overlap one another.

With a disease as complicated as Chronic Fatigue Syndrome there is no "magic bullet" to cure the disease or clear up the symptoms. Rather, a wide variety of medicines sometimes work in one situation and not in another.

Chronic Fatigue Syndrome is not an illness you can treat yourself by taking vitamins or by engaging in exercise of one type or another. (Remember: exercise may actually make it worse!) What you need is a physician who understands your problem and who will work with you. You will want to discuss the disease thoroughly with him and you may suggest that he read my other book, which gives dosages as well as detailed descriptions of drugs that I have found effective (*Chronic Fatigue Syndrome: The Struggle for Health* [CFS Institute, 500 S. Anaheim Hills Rd., Suite 128, Anaheim Hills, CA 92807. Phone 714-998-2780]).

**PHASE ZERO**  This phase involves a basic alteration of the immune system, producing decreased effectiveness of its function. This allows invasion by certain (usually viral) agents that most of us successfully fight off and develop resistance to very early in life. In other words, our immune systems begin to miss certain agents they had previously destroyed or held in check.

If a phase-zero abnormality occurs, a domino effect may ensue, triggering the other phases and affecting many bodily functions.

**PHASE I**  As a result of the decreased surveillance by the immune system that occurs in phase zero, various kinds of viral (and possibly other) infections may occur in phase I, such as:

spirochetes (such as borrelia burgdorferi—the cause of Lyme disease)
candida (if, as some propose, many symptoms are caused by an intestinal overgrowth of the yeast candida)
chlamydia
mycoplasma
protozoans
certain bacteria

Drugs that may be useful include acyclovir and low-dose alpha interferon (when used in conjunction with other drugs).

**PHASE II**   This phase further involves the immune system. Antigens—foreign substances such as viruses to which the body makes antibodies—may be abnormally dealt with at the cellular level. The result of this malfunction may be that the body's natural defense mechanisms are turned on but do not work properly.

Drugs that are sometimes effective include gamma globulin, which can produce striking effects, sometimes clearing up symptoms of this phase in a quick, dramatic, and effective fashion. Other drugs may also be helpful, including Monoamine Oxidase inhibitors, such as phenelzine (Nardil) and tranylcipromine (Parnate), which may affect the way certain white blood cells (lymphocytes) respond to antigens. Also of benefit may be cimetidine (Tagamet), ranitidine (Zantac), and other H-2 blockers, as well as doxepin (Sinequan) and other tricyclic antidepressants. Fluoxetine (Prozac) helps depression and sometimes many of the other symptoms of CFS.

**PHASE III**   The improper functioning of the immune system continues. Immune chemicals called cytokines may be produced in abnormal amounts or not at all. Ranitidine (Zantac) or cimetidine (Tagamet), drugs used to treat stomach ulcers, may also affect secretions of certain cytokines and are sometimes useful in CFS. The experimental drug Ampligen may help to correct this problem.

**PHASE IV**   Certain organs in the body, like the intestinal tract or the brain, may function improperly because their activity is affected by cytokines. Clonazepam (Klonopin) may be helpful, as might doxepin (Sinequan).

**PHASE V**   The communication between body organs is not well regulated and secondary illnesses, such as fibromyalgia, appear (see Chapter 1). This altered communication is particularly apparent when looking at brain function. Certain parts of the brain, which control the function of many of the parts of the body, may not work normally. Other drugs that affect the brain, such as the antidepressant fluoxetine (Prozac), may remedy the impaired communication between the brain and the rest of the body. If one believes that a yeast infection of the intestines can produce chemicals that could cause Chronic Fatigue Syndrome, prescribing anti-yeast diets and medications would be an appropriate Phase V treatment.

Numerous other drugs can be quite helpful in treating phases three through five, among them the calcium channel blockers, such as nimodipine (Nimotop), the anticonvulsant carbamazepine (Tegretol), or, for a yeast infection, fluconazole (Diflucan).

## CHRONIC FATIGUE SYNDROME RULES TO CONSIDER

No one treatment of Chronic Fatigue Syndrome works for everyone; treatments may lose their effectiveness over time; and multiple treatment may be necessary. You should not overexert yourself, drink alcohol, deny yourself sleep, or get into stressful situations. All of these behaviors are likely to cause relapses. Psychotherapy is helpful for dealing with stress, and acupuncture can also be of benefit for some. Naturopathic and nutritional medicine seems to help some patients as well.

## WHAT CAN YOU DO FOR SOMEONE WITH CHRONIC FATIGUE SYNDROME?

A person who has Chronic Fatigue Syndrome has, in a sense, two problems. The first is the illness. The second is dealing with it both socially and financially.

Even though Chronic Fatigue Syndrome is not life-threatening, patients are going to find their lives on hold. They sink gradually into poverty if too disabled to work. Their marriages may deteriorate. Their relationships with others may become eroded. They are going to have all kinds of medical bills to pay, especially since insurance companies are reluctant to accept the validity of Chronic Fatigue Syndrome and many refuse to pay for diagnosis or treatment.

Worst of all, their biggest problem may be getting other

people, including friends and loved ones, to believe they have something wrong with them. The tendency is for people not to offer sympathy because the patient just stays in bed and doesn't seem to do anything to help himself or herself.

Many patients report that their self-esteem and their credibility are simply destroyed by the reactions of others. They feel humiliated. They feel as though the illness is a kind of punishment and they are somehow to blame. And when they go to a nonthinking physician who suggests that the illness is in reality hypochondria, the "I told you so" or "Pull yourself together" reactions of those close to them can be devastating.

It is important to remember that the victim's life circumstances, social environment, and mental attitude did not cause the disease. If you are living with or are close to a Chronic Fatigue Syndrome patient, you must understand that he or she is not to blame for the medical problems.

Further, if you insist that the patient adopt the "right mental attitude" or "pull himself up by his bootstraps," you may further stress him or her, particularly after so many have already insinuated that the problem is imaginary.

What a person with Chronic Fatigue Syndrome needs is not criticism but support, not blame but encouragement. You can provide this by doing the following:

1. Read up on Chronic Fatigue Syndrome so you can understand the disease.
2. Encourage the patient to seek the advice of a caring physician who can help him or her.
3. Don't force the patient beyond his or her capacity. Remember, exercise can actually make the illness worse, although some exercise (just up to the point of beginning to feel fatigued) can be beneficial.
4. Remember that brain dysfunction is a part of this syndrome, so be tolerant when your friend or loved one has mood swings or cannot remember things.
5. Encourage the person to join a support group.
6. Help in any way you can. It may be cleaning house, providing meals, finding financial aid.
7. Let the person know he is valued for personal qualities, not for how much work he can perform and how entertaining

he can be. Understand that he may have an impaired sense of self-worth because he isn't as productive as he once was.

Remember, a person with Chronic Fatigue Syndrome is still a person with the same needs as anyone else but with a much-reduced ability to satisfy them.

## IS IT CONTAGIOUS?

The patient with Chronic Fatigue Syndrome probably is mildly contagious from time to time, perhaps more so at the onset. Those who attend this person are at some risk; however, the degree is not clear until we understand the disease better than we do at present.

As I mentioned, it appears that a hereditary predisposition to this disease may be necessary in order for a person to be affected with it. If that's the case, only some people are seriously at risk, and we may be able to genetically identify those people at some future time.

It may also be necessary for a virus or a toxin or both to be present for you to catch Chronic Fatigue Syndrome. Other factors such as age, sex, physical condition, stress, and so forth may play a role as well.

In short, at the present time, we cannot really say how contagious the illness may be, although it probably isn't as contagious as flu.

## CHRONIC FATIGUE SYNDROME AND THE FUTURE

In many ways the future of our understanding and treatment of Chronic Fatigue Syndrome is bright. Advances in studies of molecular biology and pharmacology as applied to virology, the brain, and the immune system are proceeding at a breath-taking rate. Although Chronic Fatigue Syndrome research in the United States has lagged because of lack of funding, more advances have been made in the last year than in all the years before.

Abroad, the Australians are making a major research effort and professionals should be seeing their reports shortly. At home there are signs that the National Institutes of Health may, at last, become involved in Chronic Fatigue Syndrome research in a meaningful and productive way and that the Centers for Disease Control is beginning to regard the disease as more than some kind of bad joke.

## THE INSURANCE DILEMMA

Disability insurance benefits are still hard to come by, since most insurance companies either delay payment for Chronic Fatigue Syndrome diagnosis and treatment or refuse it entirely. This problem may become easier as patients learn the system and the insurance companies become educated about the illness. Effective treatment exists for most patients who have access to it. (Chronic Fatigue Syndrome does resolve spontaneously in many patients after two or three years, and others improve, although they must limit their activity to avoid relapses; the first six months are usually the worst in those with an acute onset.)

The general medical community will gradually come around as well. Doctors will find themselves unable to continue to ignore the clinical presentation of the increasing parade of Chronic Fatigue Syndrome sufferers and what promises to be a significant volume of good, published research in the next few years.

I expect better treatment to be available, but not necessarily for everyone. And I would not expect a cure for Chronic Fatigue Syndrome in the near future, since treatment of the cause may require gene therapy of some sort.

As we understand the illness better, we may gain insight into possible cures by studying those who recover spontaneously. I expect the 1990s to offer more in our understanding of health and disease than all of the prior decades combined. The current rate of progress is so rapid, in fact, that I look at my own understanding of illnesses even three years ago as rather primitive and unsophisticated.

The obstacles are not primarily medical, in my view, but social, political, and economic. There is an immediate need for well-organized, unified, and well-directed Chronic Fatigue Syndrome advocacy such as exists in the AIDS movement. This advocacy is already moving forward, though slowly, through Chronic Fatigue Syndrome support groups across the country.

Overall, my conclusion is that there is great reason for optimism. True, we don't have a cure (and may not for a long time); there is little research funding; and the medical profession has yet fully to accept Chronic Fatigue Syndrome as a legitimate illness. But progress is being made on all fronts.

# 5

# Premenstrual Syndrome (PMS)

There have been few more controversial illnesses than Premenstrual Syndrome (PMS). Only a few years ago its very existence was doubted. Women with severe symptoms had to suffer silently, guiltily, thinking there was something wrong with them personally for their affliction.

Today, few doctors still doubt the existence of PMS. Yet if you go to one doctor, you'll get one treatment and, chances are, if you go to another doctor, a different treatment. Similarly, among physicians there is still no agreement whatsoever on causes of the disorder other than that functioning ovaries are required for PMS to occur. There is no test for PMS, and although the most frequently prescribed treatment (the ovarian hormone progesterone) has many advocates, most studies of this treatment have failed to show that it actually works. (Measurements of progesterone levels of women with PMS are no different than those without it.)

Thus, in many respects we are still at the beginning. The only difference is that now if you have PMS, most doctors won't tell you "It's all in your mind."

The real problem that most women face, I believe, is in getting treatment that works, as opposed to treatment that the doctor says should work but doesn't. In this chapter we look at PMS to see what may cause it. Then we'll look at some treatments you may want to discuss with your physician if your present course of treatment isn't working.

## WHAT IS PMS?

There is no real definition of the disorder that everyone completely accepts. We do, however, understand some of its biological aspects. Here's what happens: After menstruation an egg matures in the ovary. At about day 14 in the menstrual cycle, ovulation occurs. In ovulation the egg (ovum) is released from the surface of the ovary. The area of the ovary that releases the egg simultaneously begins to make progesterone and continues to do so until shortly before the onset of menstruation.

PMS occurs during this biological episode. PMS begins with ovulation (which can occur as early as day 7 of the cycle and continue until the onset of menses or, less commonly, their end). There must then be at least seven out of twenty-eight days of a marked reduction of symptoms for a syndrome to be called premenstrual. (Having the symptoms all the time would put the disorder into some other category.)

## PMS SYMPTOMS

Up to 150 symptoms of PMS have been described in the medical literature. They involve mood, behavior, and physical changes. Some of the more common are:

Depression
Irritability
Anxiety
Breast swelling and tenderness
Problems with thinking and concentration
Perceived water retention
Abdominal bloating
Fatigue
Headache
Changes in appetite
Constipation

It has been estimated that these symptoms cause some noticeable change in normal function in 40 percent of all women and severe alteration of life-style in 2 to 10 percent.

Don't confuse PMS with painful menstruation (dysmenorrhea), although the two disorders may coexist. Also, it is not necessary to have a uterus to have PMS, since women who have had hysterectomies but still have their ovaries often have the same cyclic disorder.

Probably the best way for you to diagnose PMS yourself is to keep a diary of when the symptoms occur. Recollections alone will not be accurate. If the symptoms recur with regularity around your menstrual cycle, you may very well have the disorder.

Still, when you go to the doctor be prepared for some skepticism. Your doctor may want to fit you into a more conveniently treatable cookbook illness. Even today, PMS is often misdiagnosed as any of the following disorders:

Depression
Manic-depressive disorder
Hypo- or hyperthyroidism
Diabetes
Hypoglycemia
Chronic Fatigue Syndrome
Fibroids of the uterus
Endometriosis

## DEALING WITH PMS

I describe several treatments below. If you have PMS, you will want to discuss each one with your physician. See what he or she thinks. Do they apply to you? A doctor who dismisses any or all of these therapies out of hand may simply be so old-fashioned as to dismiss PMS itself. That's the time for a new opinion.

You should also be aware of my bias. I approach PMS from a rather unique perspective as a physician who has a practice with a large number of Chronic Fatigue Syndrome patients. Virtually all women who have CFS also have severe PMS. If they had PMS before they got sick, it now has become more severe and it makes their other symptoms worse. If they never had it before, they do now. (I can think of only one of my CFS patients who doesn't.) I would even say that Chronic Fatigue Syndrome can cause PMS and that PMS is one of a spectrum of disorders that can fit under the umbrella of CFS-related ailments.

**EARLY TREATMENT** The earliest explanation of the cause of PMS was that there was an imbalance between levels of the hormones estrogen and progesterone in the body during the period after ovulation. This period is called the luteal phase, because the areas of the ovary from which the ovum was expelled is called the corpus luteum, which makes hormones until menstruation is under way.

It was thought that when the corpus luteum did not make enough progesterone women had PMS. There were, of course, many variations on this theme.

As a result, therapy consisting of supplementing progesterone (preferably with ''natural'' rather than synthetic progesterone) was thought to be the rational treatment of choice. However, since natural progesterone is digested and metabolized in the liver, it is usually not practical to take an oral preparation. (It can be taken if it is specially formulated or ''micronized.'') Women thus were given vaginal and rectal progesterone suppositories as well as progesterone pills to be placed under the tongue where they could be absorbed directly into the bloodstream.

**EFFECTIVENESS OF PROGESTERONE** Many women swear by natural progesterone, although I have read only one double-blind clinical study to support its use and then only in a specially formulated oral capsule. Further, this hormone may have the drawback of addiction. I have seen a woman who was addicted to progesterone injections (other routes being ineffective) and so felt horrible when the progesterone wore off.

The question remains: Does progesterone work? I have seen women take massive doses of progesterone, sometimes with estrogen, and have their symptoms of PMS relieved. On the other hand, I have seen other women take progesterone only to have their PMS get worse. In my own practice, since I do not know whether progesterone works in PMS, I do not prescribe it unless other treatments are ineffective.

**PROGESTERONE RECEPTORS** An alternative hypothesis is that the cause of PMS involves the effect of progesterone on its receptors (structures on the surface of cells that receive the hormone) rather than levels of progesterone per se. The relevant receptors are primarily in the brain, but are probably elsewhere, especially in the immune system, the breasts, the intestines, and the kidneys—which would help to explain the diversity of the symptoms.

Progesterone receptors affect other chemicals that transmit information and are, in turn, affected by them. The situation is very complex; some readers might prefer simply to skip over the next section. However, at least a brief awareness of this topic is necessary in order to understand the new treatments for PMS that are becoming available, with which your doctor may not yet be familiar.

**RECEPTOR PHYSIOLOGY**   A chemical transmitter such as progesterone and its receptor, which receives the chemical, are often compared to a key and a lock. The transmitter (the key) must have the proper configuration to fit into the receptor (the lock), which is usually on the surface of a cell, to cause a change in the function of the cell to occur.

If there are few receptors on the surface of the cell, they will be more sensitive and it will not take much transmitter (progesterone) to have a strong effect. Conversely, if there are many receptors available, more transmitter will be needed. The amount of available transmitter and number of receptors normally vary considerably with the rhythms of the body and also may be significantly altered if disease is present. Furthermore, if there is too much transmitter (progesterone), the actual number of receptors usually decreases (technically, down-regulation) so that overstimulation will not occur, and if there is too little transmitter, the number of receptors will increase (up-regulation).

Receptor physiology, of course, is much more involved than the brief description here, but I hope it is enough to acquaint you with these concepts.

At any rate, it has been suggested that receptors in a part of the brain called the limbic system (an area associated with emotions) might be overly sensitive to decreases in progesterone. This could cause a dysfunction of the limbic system that would manifest itself in all the symptoms we have come to call PMS. This hypothesis, or variations of it, is increasingly compelling for me.

**FURTHER UNDERSTANDING OF OVARIAN REGU-LATION**   Earlier we went through the biological steps of ovulation. Now let's take a closer look at it in a chemical way with regard to receptors.

The maturation of the ovum in the ovary is controlled by hormones. After menses begin, two hormones secreted by the pituitary gland regulate this maturation. These are called FSH (follicle-stimulating hormone) and LH (luteinizing hormone).

FSH and LH, in turn, are regulated by the amounts of estrogen in the blood, and also by another hormone called GnRH (gonadotropin releasing hormone) which comes from another area of the brain called the hypothalamus. GnRH is of special interest to us here.

Relative to PMS, secretion of the regulating hormone GnRH causes a sudden pulse of LH, which causes ovulation to occur. It also causes the corpus luteum (the area of the ovary from which the ovum is expelled) to form and secrete progesterone.

Having said that GnRH triggers a release of progesterone, let's take one step back and see what releases GnRH. The way that GnRH (as well as some other relevant hypothalamic hormones) is secreted is regulated in part by other brain chemicals (neurotransmitters). The long list of these includes beta-endorphin, one of the body's own morphine-like substances.

Other chemicals involved in regulating secretion of GnRH include serotonin, involved in mood and pain perception as well as endorphin regulation, gamma amino butyric acid (GABA), an inhibitory chemical involved in the way drugs like Xanax act to reduce anxiety, and dopamine, which can cause painful breasts and fluid retention if there is too little of it. All of these chemicals (and more) are related to hypothalamic function in the natural menstrual cycle—and also to PMS.

**ALTERATIONS IN THESE TRANSMITTERS AND TREATMENT** Putting all of the above information together, one of the leading current theories about why PMS occurs is that women with PMS have lower blood levels of beta-endorphin after ovulation than women who do not have PMS, although this finding has not been confirmed by all researchers.

It is assumed that the levels of beta-endorphin in the hypothalamus would also be low, after being normal prior to ovulation. Thus PMS may be, at least in part, a form of narcotic withdrawal, with the narcotic here the body's own.

## TREATING PMS

If your doctor wants to try progesterone for PMS, one easy method to discuss with him or her is taking oral contraceptives, which are sometimes effective. Estrogen skin patches in combination with an oral progesterone derivative taken during days 9 through 26 of the cycle have also sometimes reduced PMS symptoms.

There are a number of other medications which I believe can be effective. You may want to ask your doctor about each of them.

**NALTREXONE**   Naltrexone is a narcotic antagonist that has been used successfully to reduce the symptoms of PMS when taken on days 9 to 18 of the menstrual cycle. Seven out of ten women are reported to improve on this treatment. When naltrexone works, virtually all PMS symptoms may improve, but adverse reactions may include nausea, headache, depression, and insomnia. Using a narcotic antagonist is an application of the hypothesis that PMS may be a form of withdrawal from a morphine-like substance made by the ovaries during the first half of the cycle.

**CLONIDINE**   Clonidine is made in a skin patch and used primarily to treat high blood pressure. It decreases the secretion of norepinephrine and ameliorates these withdrawal symptoms. Actually, both naltrexone and clonidine could be given at the same time and might work more effectively, but this mode of treatment has not been reported in the medical literature. Some of my patients say that clonidine has relieved all their PMS symptoms. I have been prescribing it for several years.

**BUSPIRONE**   Buspirone (Buspar) has been reported to decrease almost all of the PMS symptoms when given during the luteal phase, so your doctor may want you to try it. Unfortunately, my patients have not usually received this benefit.

**XANAX**   Alprazolam (Xanax) produces significant reductions in anxiety, mood swings, irritability, depression, fatigue, forgetfulness, crying, cravings for sweets, abdominal bloating, abdominal cramps, and headache in PMS when it is given from day 20 through the second day of menstruation. Xanax can be addictive, a property your doctor will want to consider before prescribing it.

**BROMOCRIPTINE**   Breast tenderness can be caused by prolactin, a pituitary hormone elevated in the luteal phase. This chemical is suppressed by dopamine. Dopamine is not produced as an oral medication, but your doctor can give you bromocriptine (Parlodel), which mimics the effect of dopamine and can decrease breast tenderness and swelling. Other PMS symptoms, however, are not decreased by this medication and it also causes unacceptable nausea in many women.

**DANAZOL (DANOCRINE)**   If the nausea of bromocriptine is a problem, you may want to ask your doctor about danazol (Danocrine). This is a treatment I find useful in severe cases, and seems to be well tolerated in low doses, although it does not work for everyone. If it does work for you it will help many of the symptoms, particularly breast tenderness. It can, however, have masculinizing effects if taken for many consecutive months.

**SPIRONOLACTONE**   Spironolactone can relieve bloating in PMS and may affect other symptoms as well, including those associated with the brain. (Some researchers think that PMS may involve a degree of brain swelling. As a consequence diuretics—drugs that increase water loss—are frequently used in PMS.)

**VITAMIN B$_6$**   Some doctors use high doses of vitamin B$_6$, which acts as a catalyst in the production of certain neurotransmitters that may be deficient in PMS. A possible danger is that high doses could cause nerve damage. If your doctor suggests using B$_6$, be sure to ask about this side effect.

**MEFANEMIC ACID (PONSTEL)**   Ponstel reduces headaches, muscle aches, and fatigue. It may even help mood swings. Nonsteroidal anti-inflammatory drugs (NSAIDs) such as Ponstel or Ketoprofen (Orudis) are the treatment of choice for painful menstruation, and Ponstel and Orudis seem to have an advantage over other NSAIDs in the treatment of PMS.

**BIRTH CONTROL PILLS**  Progesterone-dominant birth control pills such as Lo-ovral also often seem to be effective. They prevent ovulation and work better than estrogen-dominant birth control pills, which may make PMS worse. Estraderm skin patches (containing estrogen) have also been used cyclically with progesterone, and subcutaneous implants have been tried with some success on an experimental basis.

**FLUOXETINE (PROZAC)**  Only modest success has been reported with the antidepressant fluoxetine (Prozac) and the appetite suppressant fenfluramine (Pondimin). Drugs that affect specific serotonin receptors are experimental and to my knowledge have not been tried in PMS yet. Medications such as Prozac, which increases serotonin levels, should be useful in women who feel depressed and crave carbohydrates, since serotonin is involved in both mood and appetite.

**VERAPAMIL, ATENOLOL, AND DOXYCYCLINE**
Other treatments that may be helpful include verapamil (Calan, Isoptin) and atenolol (Tenormin), which are usually used to treat heart and blood pressure problems. Both may also decrease anxiety, however. Curiously, doxycycline (Vibramycin), an antibiotic, may also reduce PMS. (Doxycycline was given in a double-blind study to thirty women with PMS for one month. Biopsies of the lining of the uterus revealed pathogenic microorganisms in most of them. At the end of six months all reported improvement of their PMS symptoms. A small infection of the uterus or the ovaries may be involved in PMS and, consequently, doxycycline may help. It has some immunologic benefits as well.)

**EXERCISE AND FOODS**  A natural way to treat PMS that can be somewhat effective is to increase exercise, drink extra water, avoid salty foods, and avoid caffeine (including colas and chocolate that contain caffeine).

## FUTURE TREATMENTS

Research in the area of immunology is having a direct, though limited, effect on the treatment of PMS. (The immune system is closely linked to hormonal function, although there has been little research in this area.) In the future we may have remarkable drugs that will, in various ways, work with or against the body's immune system and curtail the effects of PMS.

In addition, the ovaries make numerous substances that I have not mentioned. Perhaps one of them, so far undiscovered, is related to the cause of PMS (since strict progesterone deficiency does not appear to be responsible). I expect, however, that an interaction between the brain (especially the limbic system), the immune–hormonal system, and the ovary will ultimately be discovered to be producing PMS.

# 6
=

# Abdominal Pain and
# Gastric Problems

Perhaps no area of the body gives people as much trouble with mysterious pains and ailments as the abdominal region and stomach. Many people have a variety of abdominal problems that wax and wane, or perhaps persist lifelong, yet are seldom clearly diagnosed by their doctors.

In this chapter we are going to look at a variety of the more puzzling problems of this area of the body.

I do not intend to cover problems such as appendicitis or hemorrhoids, which any competent doctor should be able to diagnose in a thorough exam. Rather, I am going to be concerned with those gray areas that are often misdiagnosed or inadequately treated—once again, those that don't fit the cookbook. If you are concerned because you have indeterminate abdominal pain or are bloated or any of a number of other "stomach" problems and your doctor doesn't seem to be making you any better, this chapter can provide you with some insight about what could be wrong. After you read this material, you may be better able to discuss the problem with your doctor and develop a course of action that works for you.

## ABDOMINAL PAIN

Almost everyone has abdominal pain sometime. Usually, it's transitory. Then, when no specific cause can be found and the pain is short-lived, it can be attributed to a bout with the flu or distress caused by something that was recently eaten.

All abdominal pain should be considered a warning of some kind of problem. Even pain that has been going on for only a few hours can signal a serious disorder that requires immediate medical intervention. Severe abdominal pain should prompt a call to your doctor or a visit to the emergency department of your local hospital.

**IS IT SERIOUS?**   Not necessarily. However, some physicians have become so procedure-oriented that sometimes they leave common sense behind. Consider the case of Perry.

Perry had gone to his internist to complain of some problem totally unrelated to his abdominal pain. (I believe it was a fever blister on his lip.) The internist quickly took care of the complaint that had brought the young man in and then casually asked "Is there anything else at all bothering you?"

Perry thought a moment, then said "Well, I've had some stomach problems, but I don't think they're worth mentioning."

"Tell me about them," coaxed the doctor.

Perry mentioned that he had been waking up in the night with stomach distress.

"How long has this been going on?" the internist asked.

Perry replied that he couldn't really tell because he hadn't paid much attention to it, but it probably was at least two or three weeks.

"Indeed," the doctor said. Thereupon he unleashed a brief lecture on the dangers of stomach ulcers and colon cancer. He insisted that Perry immediately have both an upper and lower GI (gastrointestinal) series of X-rays.

Perry asked if maybe this was moving too far and too fast, given the fact that the tests, particularly the lower GI, were fairly uncomfortable and costly. (An upper GI involves drinking a barium solution while your esophagus and stomach are viewed by a radiologist, who looks for possible problems. A lower GI is much more distressing, involving the pumping of a barium mixture into your colon—much like an enema—and then taking photos while you attempt to hold it in.) The internist replied that it was better to be safe than sorry.

Perry wanted a second opinion, so he came to me to ask if these tests were really necessary. We talked for a while and I asked Perry about his eating habits, particularly what he ate just before he went to bed. In particular I asked if he had changed his eating habits recently.

He replied that he hadn't, except that now he was drinking a large glass of milk just before bed. He had heard that tryptophan, an amino acid, helped people to get to sleep and that milk was high in it.

I asked if the milk-drinking had started at about the same time the stomach problems had. It had. So I suggested he stop drinking milk at bedtime and report back to me.

He stopped the milk and his stomach pains immediately cleared up—without any kind of GI exam. (I'll have more to say about problems associated with milk shortly.)

**RUSHING TO FALSE CONCLUSIONS**  Thus far in this book, we have talked about doctors who perform all the usual tests only to have them come out negative and then be left with confusion instead of a diagnosis. The example of Perry is different, however, because in the case of abdominal pain I'm suggesting that a few moments of thought may help in reaching the proper solution. Sometimes the process is simple and involves taking a careful history of the patient and an analysis of his or her life-style.

While you should usually follow your doctor's advice if he says certain tests are necessary, you may first want to question him about other possibilities. Maybe something as simple as avoiding milk will be the answer. For example, could your problem be caused by:

Alcohol
Iron pills
Vitamins
Coffee or tea
Aspirin

All of the above are common stomach irritants.

**MUSCLE PAIN AS A CAUSE OF ABDOMINAL PAIN**
While ulcers, appendicitis, and numerous other disorders your doctor may consider can cause abdominal pain, there are some other causes that your doctor may have overlooked. For example, pelvic pain in women may be due to irritable bowel syndrome (see below). Abdominal pain may also be produced by a gall-bladder spasm. And then there is muscle pain.

Muscle pain is often overlooked because physicians are so accustomed to thinking that abdominal pain must come from *inside* the abdominal cavity that they do not consider that the pain may come from the muscles that enclose it (technically, myofascial pain syndrome).

One source of muscle pain that can project to the abdomen comes from the muscles along the spine in the back of the chest and lower back. Even though the pain may come from a tender spot there called a trigger point (see Chapter 1), it is felt at a distance in the abdomen. This radiation of pain to a distant location is known as referred or projected pain.

Sometimes muscle pain causes pain to be felt in the back as well as in the abdomen. I recently saw a patient who had passed one kidney stone and had no other but still complained of severe kidney pain in the back and abdomen. He had suffered for months, had been to see several urologists, and could not work. I found the appropriate trigger point in the muscles near the kidney, injected them with a concentration of salt water (normal saline), and his pain immediately went away, never to return.

If your doctor can't find a good reason for your abdominal pain, ask him to check your muscles. It may turn out that your pain is not inside your abdomen but in your muscles.

**GAS**   Everyone experiences abdominal pain caused by "gas" at one time or another. However, gas causes belching and flatulence more often than it does pain. If you complain to your doctor about these problems, he may say simply "You'll just have to live with it!" What do you do now?

There are ways to deal with the situation. But first, it's important to understand what causes gas. There are two simple causes of gas, swallowing air and the production of gas in the intestines. Let's consider each and how to get rid of them.

**Intestinal Gas**   We generate gas in our intestines as a result of bacterial metabolism, usually of undigested sugars. Sometimes these sugars cannot be digested; certain people lack the enzymes to do so. For example, people who lack the enzyme lactase, which breaks up the milk sugar lactose, cannot digest milk. If lactose passes into the large intestine undigested, it will be fermented by the bacteria that normally live there into hydrogen, methane, and carbon dioxide.

This problem is extremely common. In fact, the most common cause of excessive gas is milk intolerance due to lactase deficiency. Depending upon the efficiency of the bacteria in your colon, over a hundred quarts of gas can be made from a single quart of milk!

Of course, other sugars also produce gases. For example, beans are another common cause of gas. Beans have complex sugars that cannot be digested in the small intestine but can be metabolized by colon bacteria. There are over 200 sugars that can be metabolized that give human intestinal gas its characteristic odor. The quality and quantity of the gas depends on the type and amount of bacteria that normally live in your colon. Two other sugars which may be poorly absorbed and can cause intestinal gas are sorbitol, used in colas and other beverages, and the fruit sugar fructose.

**Getting Rid of Intestinal Gas**   Begin by eliminating the foods that can cause gas. (In too many cases the doctor has not taken the time to explain in detail what causes the gas, hence you, the patient, don't understand why the elimination of certain foods will work so well.) As already noted, milk intolerance is the main culprit. If you don't want to eliminate milk, a product called Lact-Aid, which contains lactase, can be swallowed beforehand and will help with digestion.

Another food to eliminate is beans. However, you might also consider limiting high-fiber foods, which are also a cause of gas.

When you do have gas, simethicone can be helpful. It is an ingredient found in numerous over-the-counter preparations and works by making big gas bubbles smaller.

In severe cases of gas, activated charcoal can be prescribed by your doctor. Activated charcoal is an odorless, tasteless black powder used in medicine primarily in those who have overdosed on drugs because it attaches other chemicals to it (adsorption). If needed, your doctor will probably give it to you in capsule form.

It is also possible to attack the resident bacteria that produce the gas. Much has been written about the effects of these bacteria on health and disease, but attempts to change their composition have largely failed. In my opinion, trying to change those bacteria that normally reside in your intestines is a futile effort.

Another approach is to attempt to kill the resident bacteria with antibiotics. Doctors who prescribe this technique, however, are playing Russian roulette with the patient, since the "good" bacteria that don't form gas may be killed off instead.

While you may want to discuss any or all of these methods with your doctor, eliminating foods that cause gas is the first thing to do.

**BELCHING**   Unlike the intestinal gas produced by bacteria, gas can also come from swallowing air. This produces belching (technically, aerophagy) and pain. It's important to differentiate swallowed air from intestinal gas.

Usually belching occurs because you swallow air when you eat. This phenomenon can be an exaggeration of normal swallowing and can occur during eating with the head thrust forward. Belching rarely indicates any serious disorder. Treatment usually involves training yourself to ingest less air when you eat. Just eat smaller pieces of food, chew well, and make a conscious effort not to swallow air as you do.

**CONSTIPATION**   If you have fewer than three bowel movements a week, or have to strain at eliminating a stool more than 25 percent of the time, you may be said to be constipated.

But is constipation simply the inability to eliminate? Sometimes people eliminate fairly often but still say they feel constipated.

Constipation, as a feeling, can make you quite uncomfortable. Often it produces a full or bloated feeling, although sometimes there is just a vague sensation of "unwellness." (Some gastroenterologists believe that the feeling of unwellness attributed to constipation is actually caused by a distension of the colon.) The unpleasant sensation of being constipated also may be due to release of gut chemicals called peptides into the bloodstream. These chemicals are also involved in brain function and may produce discomfort by altering the usual balance of brain peptides.

**If You Are Constipated**   If you have constipation, you should see your doctor and be sure to ask him to perform the appropriate tests. Consultation is particularly important if constipation occurs for the first time after age forty. Your doctor will probably look for a colon cancer with a sigmoidoscope, a flexible telescope that allows him to examine your colon. He can also tell if your colon muscle tone is hyperactive or slack or if there is a mass or a hard stool blocking the colon (fecal impaction). Many doctors perform sigmoidoscopies routinely in middle-aged and older patients to find growths called polyps, which can become cancerous (malignant) if not removed.

If your doctor does not do so on his own, also ask him to consider other problems, including an underactive thyroid as well as depression (particularly if you indeed feel depressed), both of which can cause constipation. If you have either of these conditions, they can be treated, and when they are the constipation usually clears right up.

**Causes of Constipation**   There are a variety of reasons why you might become constipated. We'll consider several.

**Medications.**   A great many drugs (such as codeine) can cause constipation, including some taken for high blood pressure and psychiatric problems. If you are taking any medications on a regular basis, ask your doctor whether they could be the cause. A trial period without the medication, if your doctor so advises, will allow you to see if the constipation goes away. If it does, you can ask him if there is some medication you might substitute that would not cause this side effect. Note that iron tablets or vitamins containing iron often cause constipation and very dark stools.

If you are still concerned after talking to your doctor, you can look up adverse reactions to any drug you are taking in various reference manuals. These books (such as *PDR*, the *Physician's Desk Reference*) are available from your physician or pharmacist, who will usually be glad to let you look at them. They may also be purchased at some bookstores.

**Irritable Bowel Syndrome.**   Another very common cause of constipation is irritable bowel syndrome (see below). If this is the problem, it might be treated by changing to a high fiber diet. (Although, as just noted, a high-fiber diet may contribute to intestinal gas; most therapies have both good and bad effects!)

**Rectocele.**    Rectocele is a weakening of the muscles in the rectum that can occur after childbirth and can be detected easily through a pelvic exam. With this the intestine loses some of its motility, its ability to move the contents of the bowel efficiently. This condition must be surgically corrected, although if mild, exercises to strengthen the muscles (Kegel exercises, generally used for urinary incontinence) may help. Ask your doctor.

**Anismus.**    This disorder, a spasm of the anal muscles, usually accompanies pelvic-floor muscle pain. (The pelvic floor is the layer of muscles on which the pelvic organs rest.) Anismus may be difficult for your doctor to diagnose if he is not familiar with this condition.

Some of the pelvic muscles hold the rectum at a certain angle and must relax if evacuation is to occur. If they do not relax, it may be impossible to evacuate the bowel and constipation may occur.

Anismus is also difficult to treat. If you do have it, you may want to discuss measures such as relaxation training and biofeedback with your doctor.

**Dealing with Constipation**    I usually try to deal with a patient's constipation by questioning him about bowel habits and suggesting ways to change them. Something as simple as good bowel habits can lessen the problem.

It is usually good to make a habit (condition a reflex) of having a bowel movement at a certain time of day, every day. Typically this time is after a meal, often breakfast. (A reflex that occurs after eating encourages defecation.) This conditioning gets your body used to having a bowel movement at a set time, and after a while it "wants" to.

Some people are so busy they do not like to take time to have a bowel movement, and others do not particularly like the act itself and put it off. This often adds to the constipation. Getting on schedule can reduce it.

**Fiber.**    Adding fiber to your diet can relieve constipation by adding bulk to the stool. It is thought that a certain stool weight is necessary to initiate the defecation reflex in the rectum. There are numerous bulking agents (such as Metamucil) which are mixed with water or juice. It's important to drink enough fluids with these preparations.

Green vegetables and unprocessed cereal grains, such as bran, are high in fiber.

**Water.**   One of the main functions of the large intestine is to absorb fluid in the intestinal contents. If intestinal propulsion is impaired, as it seems to be in about half of the people who suffer from constipation, more water is absorbed from the colon and stools tend to get harder. Drinking additional liquid is necessary for normal elimination whether or not you're using a fiber supplement.

**Lactulose.**   In more difficult cases I prescribe lactulose, a nondigestible sugar that comes in syrup form and can be mixed with water or other beverages. It will hold water in the intestine to keep the stool soft so that they may be more readily moved along. Lactulose has the disadvantage of other nondigestible sugars: It becomes available to the bacteria in the colon that cause gas production. The ensuing flatulence may be severe enough to discourage you from using it, but most of my patients find the relief it offers worth the inconvenience.

**Laxatives.**   It is harmful to take laxatives on more than an occasional basis, since they can damage the nerves regulating intestinal propulsion and make the situation worse and worse. Individuals who are constipated are frequently dependent on laxatives.

**Treating Constipation with Drugs**   If simpler methods fail, it is possible to treat constipation with prescription drugs, These, of course, should only be taken under direction of your doctor.

One cause of constipation may be in the peristaltic action that moves the intestinal contents along. This propulsion is controlled by nerves (the myenteric plexus). Drugs that affect nerves and relax the intestine to allow its contents to move along may be helpful. Ask your doctor about these:

**Naltrexone.** I use the drug naltrexone occasionally in severely constipated patients in whom no specific cause of constipation can be found. Naltrexone in tablet form is marketed for treating heroin addiction but sometimes works for constipation as well. Naltrexone treats constipation by blocking the effects of morphinelike chemicals made by the intestinal nerves.

There are sometimes adverse reactions to naltrexone. For someone with heart disease who has angina and needs to take a strong painkiller such as morphine, Percodan, or Demerol at a later time, naltrexone should not be used, since it will block the effects of these other drugs. Naltrexone's effects last about twenty-four hours.

**Cisapride.** Another drug that should be useful in severe constipation is not available in the United States at the time of this writing but may be approved shortly. Cisapride enhances the propulsion of food from esophagus to anus (a prokinetic effect). The drug has few adverse reactions and activates the myenteric plexus in the intestines.

Both naltrexone and cisapride are also effective treatments for a rare condition called pseudo-obstruction in which the intestines appear to be blocked but actually are not.

**PAINFUL BOWEL MOVEMENTS** If it is painful to have a bowel movement, you will be reluctant to have one. As a result you may become constipated, which could result in forming a hard stool that could make the next bowel movement even more painful. The proper course of action is to treat the cause of the pain.

The two main causes of painful bowel movements are a fissure, a laceration or cut in the anal muscle, and a thrombosed external hemorrhoid, a vein on the outside of the anus that has become clotted and swells. Internal hemorrhoids located where the end of the large intestine, the rectum, meets the anus may cause bleeding but do not usually cause pain.

Treatment of these conditions is fairly straightforward, and if you have such pain, you should see your doctor. He should be able to take steps to correct it. In the past surgery was virtually the only method of relieving hemorrhoids other than hot baths and waiting for them to go away (external hemorrhoids usually will). Today, however, besides increasing fiber in diet, the preferred nonsurgical treatment for internal hemorrhoids is to destroy them with a laser. This procedure is done under general anesthesia on an outpatient basis and is quite successful. Surgery is used only when the hemorrhoids are too large for laser destruction.

**SHARP RECTAL PAIN**  Patients sometimes complain of a sharp stabbing pain in the rectum that is not always associated with bowel movements. It can last seconds or as long as thirty minutes. This problem is embarrassing as well as uncomfortable.

Many doctors do not know how to deal with this disorder. They may suggest it has something to do with a fissure or hemorrhoids (although if you do not have either of these, this diagnosis will certainly be questionable). Alternatively, they may suggest you actually do not have the pain or that it is caused by emotional conflicts.

This pain is technically called proctalgia fugax. Estimates vary about the percentage of the population who have experienced this pain, but perhaps 10 percent have it at one time or the other. It usually occurs quite infrequently and may be best thought of as a muscle cramp.

**Treatment**  Medical treatments advocated have been varied, but the most recent one I know about is the use of the drug clonidine (Catapres), although why this drug works for this problem remains a mystery.

If you believe you have proctalgia fugax, it may be worthwhile to find a physician who will examine your anal muscles for trigger points and try to eliminate them if they are present.

**NONULCER DYSPEPSIA**  This is stomach discomfort that mimics the symptoms of an ulcer without an ulcer actually being present. One of the most common symptoms is bloat.

**Bloat**  This rather common disorder usually is defined as a vague feeling of discomfort under the breastbone, usually after eating and lasting a long time (off and on for more than four weeks), for which no specific cause could be found by your doctor. It may also involve getting full easily, feeling nauseated, and feeling that there is still food in your stomach two hours after eating.

Your doctor should be quite expert at finding the cookbook causes of these symptoms, which include:

Ulcers
Gall-bladder problems
Stomach acids backing up into the esophagus

Once your doctor has ruled out these problems, however, and the discomfort still persists, then it's time to look elsewhere.

When your doctor seems to be giving up, try suggesting the following explanations and possible courses of treatment.

**Causes of Bloated Feeling**   There is by no means universal agreement on the cause of this problem, but bloated feelings not caused by ulcers are almost always related to eating. About half the people with this problem have a delay in food leaving the stomach. Others may have a back-up of bile from the gall bladder into the stomach. Still others may have various kinds of abnormalities in stomach contraction.

Sometimes this condition is confused with irritable bowel syndrome (see below), which it is not. Bloating or nonulcer dyspepsia is related directly to food ingestion and having a feeling of delayed emptying.

Some have suggested a psychiatric component. However, studies have shown that people without any kind of detectable psychiatric disorder still have this problem.

The situation has been further complicated by the discovery that a bacterium called Helicobacter pylori may actually cause ulcers. Although not much has been written in the medical literature so far about this bacterium as a cause of nonulcer dyspepsia, some authorities believe it to be one. These bacteria can be treated with antibiotics and bismuth. Your doctor may want to try this course of action to see if it works for you.

**Treating Nonulcer Dyspepsia**   I have found the following method quite effective. My general approach to this problem with my patients is to treat it just as if it were an ulcer or an inflamed stomach. I prescribe antacids or H-2 blockers that decrease stomach acid production. In addition, I prohibit alcohol, tobacco, and certain drugs, particularly those related to aspirin, which can irritate the lining of the stomach.

Usually this works.

If it does not, you should consider asking your doctor about having an endoscopic exam that uses a thin flexible telescope to look into the stomach to see if something else is amiss. Maybe there is an ulcer that is not healing. Is the outlet of your stomach scarred? In short, if after treatment the problem does not resolve, you probably should have a visual examination of your stomach. If your doctor suggests doing an upper-GI X-ray instead of endoscopy, remember that the X-ray is much less sensitive at detecting ulcers.

If the visual exam or endoscopy (with a biopsy to see what suspicious tissue may really be) is normal, talk to your doctor about two medications which he may not be using. A drug called cisapride (already mentioned as a treatment for constipation) may help in some cases when it becomes available in the United States. The antibiotic erythromycin may also help the stomach to empty more rapidly. Another currently available drug that may enhance stomach-emptying is metoclopramide (Reglan), used primarily to reduce nausea. It has adverse reactions, however, which may limit your doctor's ability to prescribe it for you.

**FALSE GALL-BLADDER ATTACK**   Yet another source of confusing abdominal pain is a false gall-bladder attack (biliary dyskinesia). A problem with the nerves regulating gall-bladder movement can result in a painful spasm of the gall-bladder muscle. This condition mimics a true gall bladder attack.

Biliary dyskinesias can sometimes be treated with such medications as Valium, Xanax, and Klonopin.

A true gall-bladder attack is caused by stones in an inflamed gall bladder. The pain can be excruciating. Your doctor should be quite competent at diagnosing this problem (called acute cholecystitis) and treating it in a variety of ways. (There are even nonsurgical techniques in use today that break up the gallstones with sound waves.) The gall bladder may be inflamed without gallstones being present. This condition may be diagnosed by examining the bile obtained during endoscopy.

## HEARTBURN     (GASTROESOPHAGEAL     REFLUX)

Heartburn is a burning sensation behind the breastbone that may go up into the throat. It sometimes radiates into the back and may be felt where the stomach is, below the tip of your breastbone. It can cause a very severe pain and may be confused with peptic ulcer disease. It can also be confused with angina (see Chapter 8), mitral valve prolapse, or irritable bowel syndrome. It is made worse by overeating, lying on the back, bending over, smoking, obesity, drinking alcohol, eating spicy foods, or taking aspirin.

The best description of typical heartburn I have read compares the stomach and the esophagus to a teapot. In his book *Gut Reactions*, Dr. W. Grant Thompson describes a stomach full of food and acid tipping over and emptying into a spout (esophagus) when a person lies down or bends over.

If you have this type of pain, you should indeed see a doctor to be sure it is not angina or mitral valve prolapse. A technique some doctors use to determine the difference quickly is to give you some antacid or Gaviscon, another antacid that foams into the junction of your stomach and esophagus. The pain will usually decrease if it is due to heartburn. Chest pain should be carefully evaluated by your doctor.

**What Causes Heartburn?**     Many times people equate having a hiatus hernia (a bulging of part of the stomach into the chest through a hole in the diaphragm) with having heartburn. Having a hiatus hernia does not mean you have heartburn or vice versa. A person can have a hiatus hernia without heartburn. Hiatus hernia that causes no symptoms, in fact, is quite common.

Heartburn is usually caused by stomach acid that moves back up your esophagus (gastroesophageal reflux). Reflux usually occurs because of a loosening of the lower sphincter muscle between the esophagus and the stomach, which is supposed to stay closed when one is not swallowing.

**Misdiagnosing Heartburn**     I have frequently seen patients with this problem after they had been to see cardiologists for severe chest pain they thought might be a heart attack. Many even had radiation of the pain to the neck and left arm.

After a heart problem had been ruled out, they were sent on their way with no diagnosis or treatment, as if the cardiologist felt that since the pain was not caused by the heart it was of no further concern.

On the other hand, sometimes a doctor will misdiagnose reflux as asthma. Some people wake up in the night choking or short of breath. If your doctor doesn't realize that the problem is caused by stomach acid in the esophagus, he might treat you for asthma. But asthma medicine relaxes the esophageal muscle and can worsen heartburn.

Reflux can actually make asthma worse. If reflux is severe, acid may actually spill over from the esophagus into the throat and down into the lungs during sleep. This condition, called aspiration, may worsen preexisting asthma. Aspiration may harm the lungs and acid in the esophagus may make asthma worse. Patients with this sort of reflux may also complain of hoarseness.

Mild heartburn does not require much testing. Your doctor may be able to diagnose it by giving you antacids to see if this makes an immediate difference. He may also recommend an X-ray of your esophagus or an endoscopy. These tests are a good idea because your esophagus could be burned and scarred or precancerous changes could take place from constant acid burn.

**Heartburn Treatment**   Since the basic cause of heartburn is stomach acids in the esophagus, the first order of treatment is to neutralize those acids. Your doctor will probably give you antacids. If you do not respond, he may want to use drugs that decrease acid secretion such as ranitidine (Zantac).

A good sleeping position is also vital. It is important to sleep with the head of the bed up on blocks or telephone books (not with just your head elevated on pillows, because this position will only jackknife your stomach and possibly make the problem worse). With the bed elevated, the ''teapot'' won't empty all night and burn your esophagus.

Many doctors fail to tell patients about this change in sleeping position, and just as many fail to warn them about the side effects of drugs that can loosen the lower esophageal sphincter.

Some authorities believe that the best long-term way to treat this problem is by getting food out of your stomach rapidly so that the stomach distension won't cause acid to spill over. Emptying the stomach more rapidly can be aided by certain medications. The only one of these currently marketed in the United States is metoclopramide (Reglan). Reglan works well, but adverse reactions are fairly common.

One drug you should ask your doctor about is sucralfate (Carafate), which can coat the esophagus and greatly reduce the pain. Crush it and mix it with water (sucralfate liquid is not yet available in this country) and take it fifteen minutes before meals.

If other medications are ineffective, ask your doctor about omeprazole (Prilosec), which almost completely cuts out gastric-acid secretion. At the present time, Prilosec is only approved for use for thirty to sixty days. This period of time, however, may be long enough to allow your esophagus to heal.

**Surgery to Help Heartburn**   If all else fails, surgery sometimes works by tightening the lower esophageal sphincter. It is recommended in 5 to 10 percent of the cases. If this course of action is recommended to you, first have a careful evaluation of your esophagus to rule out other disorders.

If you have achalasia (a tightening of the lower esophagus that won't let food go down), scleroderma (a thickening and loss of pliability of the esophagus), or esophageal spasm (in which the esophagus goes into painful contractions), you do NOT want this operation. The operation can make your lower esophageal sphincter so tight that it will be hard for you to swallow and you will have esophageal bloat, which is extremely uncomfortable.

In addition, an antireflux procedure is a major operation and is technically difficult to perform. Sometimes such surgery fails and must be repeated.

**Drugs to Avoid**   Certain medications can make heartburn worse. You should avoid them if possible: Ask your doctor if you can switch to a different medication. They include oral contraceptives (progesterone), aspirin, and other nonsteroidal anti-inflammatory drugs (Motrin, Naprosyn, Feldene, etc.); tricyclic antidepressants; phenothiazines (used to treat schizophrenia); theophylline (used to treat asthma); caffeine (related to theophylline); calcium channel blockers; any anticholinergic; and asthma drugs such as terbutaline (Brethine).

More and more doctors are learning about acid in the esophagus as a cause of chest pain. Ten years ago I saw many patients with this disorder improperly diagnosed and treated. Five years ago I still saw quite a few, now even fewer. There are still, nevertheless, those who are mistreated or not treated at all.

## SWALLOWING PROBLEMS

Now let's consider another digestive-system problem some people experience: difficulty in swallowing.

Any time you have a problem swallowing (dysphagia), you need to have a medical evaluation. Difficulty in swallowing does not usually relate to any psychological problem, so you should be reluctant to accept such a diagnosis. Swallowing problems can arise from any of several causes. Most can usually be discovered by careful examination by your doctor.

An important distinction the physician should make is whether the difficulty is just with solid food or with both liquids and solids. Solid-food problems suggest an obstruction in the esophagus (a mechanical disorder). Difficulty swallowing both solids and liquids is usually a motor disorder, meaning that there's something amiss with your ability to control the muscles involved in swallowing. If your problem is mechanical, your doctor may proceed to treat it directly. If, however, it is a motor problem, a different form of treatment is required.

Another important distinction is whether it is hard for you to *initiate* a swallow or whether the problem occurs *after* you start to swallow. In the throat and upper third of the esophagus, the type of muscle is called skeletal and is the same type of muscle that moves the bones of your body. The rest of the way down the esophagus is smooth muscle, like that of your intestines. Different types of diseases affect these different kinds of muscles. Defining where the problem takes place will greatly help your doctor to understand and treat it.

If you have trouble swallowing, your doctor should order an X-ray of your esophagus. This procedure involves the swallowing of thick barium and reveals obstructions or mechanical disorders almost all the time. It also usually reveals motor disorders.

Another test your doctor may need to do is called manometry, in which pressures are measured in your esophagus. Manometry may reveal a motor disorder and, combined with use of a device that measures acidity in the lower esophagus, can also help diagnose a backing up of acids from the stomach into the esophagus.

Treatment is still not very good. Until quite recently, it was thought that using drugs like calcium channel blockers, particularly diltiazem (Cardizem) or other smooth-muscle relaxant drugs such as nitroglycerin, would keep the esophagus from going into spasm (just as they do in the arteries of the heart to prevent angina). It was hoped that this antispasmodic effect would aid swallowing.

Although they still may be worth a try, most studies thus far have not demonstrated a benefit, especially in reducing the production of pain. You may want to ask your doctor about the drug trazodone (Desyrel), used primarily as an antidepressant. It may occasionally help esophageal spasm and could be prescribed in a resistant case.

## IRRITABLE BOWEL SYNDROME

This diagnosis is frequently made when you have abdominal pain, diarrhea, and constipation and no obvious cause can be found. For many doctors, however, irritable bowel syndrome suggests that the problem really isn't in your gut but in your head. In fact, many physicians believe that it is the more neurotic or psychologically disturbed patients who will tend to complain of irritable bowel syndrome. Unfortunately, this belief on your doctor's part will do nothing to help you.

Take some comfort in the fact that irritable bowel syndrome is real and probably 20 percent of the population suffers from it. It can be uncomfortable. But there are ways of successfully treating irritable bowel syndrome, and once you recognize that it is a legitimate illness, you often can move forward to recovery.

The remainder of this chapter identifies irritable bowel syndrome, gives some idea of what causes it, and then looks at current methods of dealing with it. If your doctor has arrived at this diagnosis for you, you may want to read this material very carefully and discuss some of the treatments suggested near the end.

If you are over fifty or have blood in your stool, your doctor should examine your colon using procedures such as colonoscopy or sigmoidoscopy, and/or a barium enema (lower GI), an X-ray of the colon. These tests are done to rule out more serious problems such as cancer or colitis, which is an inflammation of the colon. A blood test can check for anemia and inflammation.

**WHAT IS IRRITABLE BOWEL SYNDROME?** The most common symptoms of this disorder are alternating diarrhea and constipation. There is often abdominal pain, which may be relieved by passing gas or by having a bowel movement. Other symptoms are stomach rumbling, gas, a sensation that you have not completely emptied after a bowel movement, and small, hard stools at times. Occasionally there may be related complaints involving the bladder, as well as gynecological symptoms (possibly caused from the intestines), colds, back and joint pain, allergies, and headaches.

Many people also complain of having the feeling of a lump in their throat. (Not too many years ago all the people who complained of such lumps in their throats were thought to have psychiatric problems and the disorder was actually given the name globus hystericus.)

There is said to be no relationship between irritable bowel syndrome and globus. However, I have treated people with globus in the same way as those with heartburn, in whom acid from the stomach goes into the esophagus and burns it, and their globus problem went away. Globus may also be caused by contraction of the throat muscles and may be related to stress. In these cases it responds well to antidepressants.

**WHAT CAUSES IRRITABLE BOWEL SYNDROME?** A great many factors could be involved in producing the symptoms. Let's begin by looking at them historically.

**Spastic Colon** The various symptoms of irritable bowel syndrome have led doctors to search for causes in the gall bladder, the stomach (ulcers), and elsewhere. Typically, tests will all come back negative. This led to some interesting diagnoses, especially spastic colon. If you had irritable bowel syndrome when you were a child, you probably remember the term *spastic colon*, which is still used to some extent today.

No one seemed to know what to do about the spastic colon, although there was general agreement that the symptoms were caused by intestinal spasms, particularly of the large intestine, that could cause pain and constipation, and perhaps diarrhea if the spasms relaxed for some unknown reason. Treatment involved medication that blocked the nerves that controlled the intestinal muscles. It helped a little. Psychotherapy and hypnosis may also have been suggested because the doctor frequently assumed spastic colon was a psychological disorder. (They may also actually help somewhat.)

**Fiber** In the early 1970s a new answer was discovered. Denis Burkitt, a British doctor working in Africa who had already become famous by having a disease named after him (Burkitt's lymphoma, a lymph-node cancer found mainly in Africa), found that natives living in the bush and eating a diet of a lot of raw vegetables high in fiber, did not seem to have irritable bowel syndrome (or several other colonic disorders, for that matter).

The conclusion was drawn that irritable bowel syndrome was caused by the fact that in our modern society we did not eat enough fiber. Almost immediately, eating a high-fiber diet became popular in the United States. This change was even more remarkable since prior to this time most doctors used to recommend the exact opposite to their patients: less fiber, not more.

Of course, the big question is: Does fiber work? Believe it or not, after twenty years of research there is no definitive proof one way or another whether increased fiber helps irritable bowel syndrome. (An article in *Gastroenterology* in 1990 compared giving fiber and placebo cookies to patients suffering from irritable bowel syndrome in a controlled crossover study—usually the most precise kind—and found *both* treatments equally effective.)

You can try fiber. If it works for you, good. If not, read on. High fiber diets are beneficial in general health maintenance. They may decrease the incidence of colon cancer, although some authorities regard this notion as overly simplistic.

**Lower Pain Threshold**    Some patients have an above-normal genetic susceptibility to pain. In other words, you may be genetically built to feel your pain at a lower threshold than the rest of the population. Your gut may be normal, but it feels abnormal.

This phenomenon of genetic pain thresholds is well documented. It is best illustrated by silent heart attacks (technically, silent myocardial ischemia). In these cases a decrease in blood flow to the heart muscle should cause angina, but the person affected does not feel any chest pain. These people have a higher-than-normal pain threshold. Higher or lower thresholds to pain can be extremely difficult for doctors to diagnose and to deal with.

**Parasites**    If your major symptom is chronic diarrhea, tests may suggest the presence of a parasite, perhaps caused by a tiny creature often contracted while traveling outside the United States. Workers from Third World countries may spread parasites in the United States.

Irritable bowel patients I have treated for giardia, a tenacious parasite sometimes found in mountain streams, with a medication called metronidazole (Flagyl) have found that their irritable bowel syndrome completely cleared up.

The parasite blastocystis may cause diarrhea, and can also be treated by using Flagyl. This drug sometimes has some side effects, such as nausea, headache, and diarrhea, but I believe the potential benefits usually outweigh the risks.

**Food Intolerance**    Your irritable bowel syndrome may occasionally be caused by a food intolerance that does not necessarily have to be an allergy. You simply may not be able to digest certain foods. You may want to eliminate certain foods from your diet to see if the problem clears up. Here is the usual suspect list:

Milk
Eggs
Corn
Wheat
Citrus fruit

Some people with irritable bowel syndrome will lack the enzyme lactase, which digests the sugar lactose, found in milk (discussed at the beginning of this chapter). Eliminating all milk products should eliminate symptoms if lactase deficiency is the cause of your problem.

**Irritable Bowel Syndrome and Chronic Fatigue Syndrome**   The problem could be caused by Chronic Fatigue Syndrome. Almost all CFS patients have irritable bowel syndrome, often quite severely. The good news is that clearing up their Chronic Fatigue Syndrome clears up the irritable bowel syndrome (see Chapter 4).

**Yeast Infections**   After the publication of *The Yeast Connection*, by William G. Crook, M.D., and other books damning yeast for virtually all maladies, many people began to feel that yeast causes irritable bowel syndrome. I don't think it commonly does.

I am willing to look for a yeast connection and will sometimes do lab tests to try to prove this diagnosis. But I have not yet found one case where a yeast infection that I could identify caused irritable bowel syndrome. Patients occasionally respond to antiyeast medication, however. I am hoping that studies on yeast causing irritable bowel syndrome will soon appear in the medical literature.

**Hyperactive Gut**   Today we still believe that irritable bowel syndrome is often related to a dysfunction of the intestines. If you have the problem, probably your gut is overly sensitive to certain stimuli, altering how the intestinal nerves communicate information. The intestinal nervous system is very complex and is similar in its function to the brain. The same transmitter chemicals are present in both systems. It is not unreasonable to suspect that some of these chemicals are dysregulated in the intestines and possibly the brain as well.

**TREATING YOUR IRRITABLE BOWEL**   A wide variety of treatments for irritable bowel syndrome exists. Often therapy is a matter of trial and error and then sticking with whatever works. As noted, fiber may help in some cases. I still advise fifteen to twenty grams a day of fiber for many patients with this problem. (My mother-in-law bakes bran cookies for me; I have them every morning and they seem to be working!)

You may also want to ask your doctor about the following medications, which can prove to be helpful.

Loperamide (Imodium) has been helpful for those people who have painless diarrhea or alternating diarrhea and constipation with pain. (Those with alternating diarrhea and constipation without pain had no improvement or got worse.)

Loperamide, however, is a narcotic and, like codeine, can itself cause constipation. However, loperamide does not get into the brain and so cannot cause addiction. As a result, you can buy it over the counter.

I have also been using antidepressants to treat irritable bowel syndrome since 1968. These drugs seem to be effective whether you are depressed or not. The older antidepressants work better if you have diarrhea. Newer ones, such as fluoxetine (Prozac), may work on constipation also.

Then there is the matter of hormones. The most spectacular results I have seen in the treatment of irritable bowel syndrome have involved the synthetic hormone leuprolide acetate (Lupron).

Thinking that pituitary and ovarian hormones might be involved in the cause of this problem (since it is worse premenstrually and occurs more often in women than in men), researchers gave Lupron, which decreases the secretion of pituitary hormones which affect the ovary, to five women with incapacitating irritable bowel syndrome.

All of them responded marvelously. One of them had no ovaries or uterus, suggesting that Lupron works directly on the gut as well. When it was stopped they relapsed. Treatment with Lupron is being used more widely in severe cases and is something you should definitely ask your doctor about. Be aware, however, that this is a very new method of treatment and large-scale experiments, although under way, have not been published yet. Lupron, as you might expect, is being tried in severe PMS.

# 7
=

# Impotence and Prostate Problems

A man with no apparent medical problems who went to his doctor complaining of problems with erection used to be given a shot of the male hormone testosterone. Sometimes the doctor didn't care whether or not the fellow had sufficient levels of the hormone already in his blood; the only remedy was the shot. If that did not help him he was told he had to live with it or see a psychiatrist. This form of treatment was very common as recently as ten years ago.

If the man went to a psychiatrist or psychologist (there were no ''sexual therapists'' then), he was likely to have insight-oriented psychotherapy of the Freudian kind, which hardly ever helped. If the therapist happened to be on the cutting edge he might use the Masters and Johnson techniques. Either way, the fellow was told that about 90 percent of impotence was in his mind and had to be treated with some sort of psychobehavior therapy. There was no other recourse.

Today the outlook is far different. We have discovered that there are many physical disorders causing impotence that can be successfully treated. In fact, probably more than half of impotent men are in this category.

Unfortunately, some doctors are still living in the Dark Ages. If your doctor only wants to give you a testosterone shot or says it's all in your head, consider the other therapies discussed below.

In this section I give a brief description of certain psychological techniques that have been found effective. Then I discuss the organic aspect and suggest remedies your doctor may not have mentioned. My goal is to present an overview of what's currently happening in this rapidly changing field. Too often a physician gives a quick and inadequate explanation and then leaves you to wonder and hope. If you're not getting better, this information may allow you to ask some pointed questions and possibly to find some help.

At the end of the chapter we discuss some common prostate disorders and how they are diagnosed and treated.

**SEXUAL THERAPY**   During the 1970s many doctors assumed that performance anxiety or a related difficulty was the primary cause of failure to get or sustain an erection. Most men have experienced this at some time. Worrying about performing can worsen the situation.

Many sexual therapy techniques have been developed; to describe them is beyond the scope of this book. Suffice it to say that they can be found in the psychology section of most bookstores, and these techniques are still very helpful to those impotent men who are considered to have their erectile dysfunction (the preferred term) caused by performance anxiety.

At one time sexual therapy was regarded as a rather straightforward matter of heightening sexual arousal while decreasing sexual anxiety.

**STRESS**   Today we realize that some impotence is transient, related to a life situation: stress, problems between partners, fatigue, guilt about a sexual liaison, illness, or something similar.

To determine if a life situation is the cause, you should consider whether the erectile problem occurred suddenly. If it came about at roughly the same time as a stressful situation, the obvious solution is to attempt to resolve the stressful problem. When that is done, the impotence usually will likewise disappear. Short-term cognitive counseling stressing problem-solving often helps.

**DISEASES THAT ADVERSELY AFFECT ERECTIONS**

In addition to worry about getting an erection (performance anxiety), a variety of diseases can cause impotence. But first it is important to understand how an erection occurs.

Basically, the penis becomes rigid when the muscles that regulate the diameter of the arteries in two chambers in its shaft (the corpora cavernosa) relax so that the chambers can fill with blood. Anything that interferes with this process will prevent an erection.

It has long been realized that there are some diseases which do just that, usually by affecting nerves. They include:

Diabetes
Prostate problems
Alcoholism
Multiple sclerosis
Severe arterial disease (which blocks the flow of blood into the legs and the penis as well)

Your doctor should be able to examine you for these disorders and determine if they are a factor. If he hasn't, ask him about them.

**MEDICATIONS THAT ADVERSELY AFFECT ERECTIONS**  In the 1970s we began to realize that many medications could cause erectile difficulties, and it may be useful to list some of them here. Most of these drugs either interfere with nerve transmission, reduce blood flow required for erection, interfere with the effects of male hormones, or affect the brain. If you are taking one of these medications, ask your doctor if you can switch to something else to see whether eliminating the drug will also solve the potency problem.

*High blood pressure pills.* Almost every drug used to treat high blood pressure has been reported to cause impotence. Exceptions are minoxidil (Loniten), known better to the public as a lotion to treat baldness, and drugs called angiotensin-converting-enzyme inhibitors. Calcium channel blockers may not have this effect, either.

*Every psychotropic drug* I can think of, except perhaps the benzodiazepines (Valium, Xanax, and the like), has been reported to cause erectile dysfunction, some more than others.

*Chronic substance abuse* of almost all kinds (including nicotine, which constricts arteries) can cause impotence. Impotence is so common among heroin abusers that I was impelled to try a new treatment that I discuss later.

*Drugs that affect hormonal function,* including cimetidine (Tagamet), digoxin, and ketoconazole (Nizoral), affect erection.

**MEASURING IMPOTENCE**   It's important to determine if your impotence is organic or psychogenic (psychological). The basic technique involves measuring erections while you sleep (nocturnal penile tumescence). The results will help your doctor prescribe the appropriate treatment.

Men naturally get erections when they sleep. While these are not related to actual sexual stimulation, the mechanism of this erection is presumed to be similar to sexually stimulated erection. If a man had normal erections while sleeping but could not get an erection during intercourse, it would obviously suggest some psychological problem. On the other hand, an inability to get an erection during sleep would indicate organic impotence.

Measuring erections is difficult, however, and also can be affected by sleep disorders. To determine erection, a measurement must be made of penile circumference and rigidity. Simple methods once used, like the stamp test (wrapping perforated strips of stamps around the penis to see if they were broken in the morning), are no longer considered reliable. Today a computerized monitoring device called a RigiScan is frequently used.

This procedure often determines quickly whether the problem is organic or psychogenic and then treatment can be appropriately prescribed.

**TREATING ORGANIC IMPOTENCE WITH TESTOS-TERONE**   Treatment for organic impotence with testosterone is often not appropriate. Hormonal causes of impotence are uncommon and probably represent only around 10 percent of all cases. However, because many men are concerned about possible hormone deficiency, I will discuss it further.

Testosterone is the primary male hormone. It is necessary for adequate libido and ejaculation, but not for erection. In men deficient in testosterone, night erections are suppressed but erection in response to erotic films may not be.

No one is exactly sure what level of testosterone is necessary in each individual for sexual function. Hence, if your doctor gives you an injection, it's literally a shot in the dark. As a consequence, giving testosterone injections for sexual dysfunction can be much like giving $B_{12}$ shots—a placebo.

If your doctor insists on giving you one, it may help. But the benefit may come simply from the fact that you think it will.

**MEDICATIONS FOR TREATING IMPOTENCE**  Some medications may be helpful in treating impotence. If you're having a potency problem, you will want to consider each of the ones we discuss here and then bring it up for discussion with your doctor. One or more may be helpful to you.

Naltrexone, a narcotic antagonist (it works to block the effects of a narcotic) may help if there is a psychogenic (psychological) problem. Brain levels of narcotic chemicals produced in the body may be too high in some patients and inhibit sexual desire and erection.

Yohimbine (Yocon) was used years ago in an arcane medication called Latrodex that also had such unusual and potentially deadly ingredients as strychnine and nux vomica. Yohimbine alone, however, is the only oral agent other than naltrexone that has been shown to be effective in a double-blind trial concerned with psychogenic impotence. It does not work in organic impotence.

Papaverine is a medication injected into the tissue of the penis that fills with blood during an erection and dilates its smooth muscles. Papaverine will cause an erection regardless of the cause of the dysfunction. An obvious deterrent is the injection site.

Nitroglycerin paste, the medication used in cardiac angina treatment, is being tried to induce erections. It is applied to the penis as an artery dilator. Interestingly, it works on increasing erections induced by erotic films. It is absorbed by the vaginal tissues during intercourse and may give the woman a headache from dilation of the arteries in her brain.

**PROSTHESES**  Recently a wide variety of mechanical devices (prostheses) that can be implanted have come into widespread use. Some provide a permanent rigidity; other devices allow the penis to become erect or flaccid at will. These prostheses have been widely accepted, but they can have adverse physical and psychological effects. Discuss this option thoroughly with your urologist before attempting to use a prosthesis.

**FEMALE LIBIDO**   Some men who experience impotence blame it on a lack of interest in their partners. These men say that their female partners don't have enough sexual desire and that the disinterest is caused by a lack of female hormones.

The medical facts do not support this argument. Female libido does not seem to be hormonally regulated, so far as can be determined by blood levels. A group of psychologically normal women with normal libido were selected and their relevant hormones measured through the menstrual cycle. There was no relationship between hormonal levels and libido, so it would not be possible for a lack of hormones to cause a lack of desire.

Unfortunately, however, our treatment and understanding of both decreased libido and production of orgasm are some of the most poorly understood of all aspects of human sexuality.

At the same time, the study of impotence is increasing in scope. Research is discovering what chemicals cause the muscles that regulate the penis to relax, thus allowing the caverns in the penis to fill with blood. As these chemicals are determined, medications that mimic their effect can be developed to correct impotence "on the spot."

Since the brain is obviously involved in erection, oral drugs that would have an effect on both the penis and the brain are being investigated. Recent work has also suggested that some patients cannot close off their penile veins appropriately so blood cannot be stored in the penis and they are unable to maintain erections. This condition may be surgically corrected by tying off veins which drain blood from the penis. Those who cannot obtain an erection because of inadequate flow of blood through penile arteries may be improved by surgery, as well.

## PRIAPISM

This condition, inability to lose an erection, though rare, can be serious as well as uncomfortable, since gangrene of the penis can occur if blood flow in and out stops, as it essentially does in an erection. In this situation an erection will not go down (or detumesce). Priapism can occur with some treatments for impotence. Its occurrence generates an emergency.

Priapism can be treated by injection into the penis of substances that cause it to become flaccid or by vascular surgery.

One antidepressant, trazodone (Desyrel), has been reported actually to cause priapism. On the other hand, this adverse reaction may be used therapeutically in the proper dosage to treat impotence.

## PROSTATE PROBLEMS

The prostate is a walnut-sized gland located just beneath the male bladder. Its site is an area between the anus and the scrotum called the perineum. The testicles connect to the prostate, which provides secretions during ejaculation.

Prostate problems occasionally cause impotence. At one time or another during his life, almost every man will have a problem with his prostate. Such problems can take many forms and have a variety of causes.

The most common prostate problems are difficulty in urination, painful urination, inability to achieve or maintain an erection, and, occasionally, blockage of the urethra that makes urination impossible. These symptoms can be accompanied by lower back pain as well as a fullness in the lower abdomen. An infected prostate can produce the sensation of sitting on a hot walnut. In some cases of prostate infection fever, chills, and generalized illness may develop.

Prostate treatment was woefully inadequate in the past. Urologists seldom prescribed antibiotics because the prostate has a kind of barrier that resists the penetration of such drugs unless acutely infected. Surgery was therefore sometimes necessary.

If a milder, longer-lasting chronic infection was present, physicians would simply tell men that they would have to live with it. As a result, the infection would sometimes result in abscesses and the need for surgery.

The Centers for Disease Control noted the underprescription of medication for prostate problems several years ago, which helped to correct this deficiency. More recently urologists may in fact have been overprescribing antibiotics.

**CORRECT TREATMENT** An early method of treating a chronic inflammation of the prostate, whether caused by bac-

terial infection or not, that is still effectively used is prostate
massage. In this therapy the physician inserts his gloved finger into the anal canal until he can feel the prostate through
the wall of the colon. He then applies pressure, typically
from the sides toward the center, until surplus prostatic fluid
has been expelled into the bladder or out through the penis.
The prostate massage can be extremely painful and has been
described as the male counterpart to the pain experienced by
women during birth. (Of course, the massage only lasts a
few seconds.)

Massaging the prostate also has an addictive feature. The
prostate tends to become used to the massage and in some
cases will not dispel prostatic fluid in the normal manner, thus
requiring massages on a regular basis.

You should be careful about having a physician apply pressure to the prostate unless there is sufficient reason to warrant
it. (I have heard of some doctors who regularly massage a
male's prostate whenever there is a complaint of lower back
pain even though that pain may be caused by muscle spasms
of the back or by lumbar nerve problems.)

The more appropriate treatment for both bacterial and abacterial prostate problems has been a combination of antibiotics
and prostate massage. (In England the standard practice is the
prescription of antibiotics alone. Perhaps as a result, the number of prostate surgeries required there is higher than in the
United States.)

**TYPES OF PROSTATE PROBLEMS**     There are at least
six common disorders of the prostate. It's important to determine which one you have, since treatments vary depending on
the cause.

**1. Acute Prostatitis (Bacterial)**     This ailment is not hard
for your doctor to diagnose and treat. You will usually have
severe pain, high fever, signs of a urinary infection, feel horrible, and your prostate will be extremely tender when palpated
(felt) during rectal exam. Your doctor should give you antibiotics—in extreme cases, intravenously. Antibiotics are usually hard to get into the prostate, but when it is severely
inflamed they penetrate well.

**2. Chronic Prostatitis (Bacterial)**  This disorder causes less severe symptoms than the acute condition but will still usually produce a tender prostate, recurrent urine infections, and signs of prostate infection. (The urologist can express some prostatic fluid on a slide during a massage and can examine it quickly for infection. A urine sample would also show chronic prostatitis if it is obtained after a prostate massage.)

Treatment of chronic bacterial prostatitis can require taking antibiotics over a long period of time. The most effective drugs include Bactrim (Septra), which can get past the prostate barrier. Newer drugs, such as Noroxin or Cipro can be even more effective.

Sometimes specific bacteria or other microorganisms are found or suspected, and different antibiotics may be required. Treatment often must continue for months or the infection will return. Sometimes doctors prescribe too brief a duration of treatment such as ten days or so. If your problem recurs, you may want to ask your doctor if you should take your medication for a longer period.

**3. Chronic Abacterial Prostatitis**  No infection is found in this disorder, although signs of inflammation (white blood cells) are seen in the urine. The symptoms are fairly similar to chronic bacterial prostatitis, but the condition does not respond well to antibiotics although they are usually tried, since bacteria are sometimes not easily detected and the usual supposition is that there may be a bacterial cause for the problem.

Abacterial prostatitis may be the result of urine with or without bacteria going into the prostate. Without going into great anatomic detail, the muscles of part of the urethra (the tube that urine goes through from the bladder through the prostate and into the penis) may spasm, causing a backflow of urine into the prostate. This dysfunction, as well as other prostate conditions, can radiate pain into the testicles and the end of the urethra.

Medications to relax the part of the urethra that is in spasm are often successful. Although Prazosin (Minipress) and terazosin (Hytrin) are usually given to treat high blood pressure, they often work dramatically to reduce urethral spasm. Another technique is the use of a low dose of estrogen for two or three weeks. Diethylstilbestrol, a form of estrogen, has been used; if it helps, it can be continued indefinitely. "The treatment is simple, inexpensive, harmless, and effective," wrote the author of one study using this drug.

**4. Prostatodynia (Prostatosis)**    Patients with this disorder have the same symptoms as with abacterial prostatitis, but no white blood cells are found. If no signs of inflammation are present your doctor may begin to think you have psychological problems. If you do, it may be unclear whether the psychological problems are a cause of the prostatodynia or are caused by the disorder. Treatment may be the same as for abacterial prostatitis, except that psychological counseling also may be in order.

**5. Enlargement of the Prostate (Benign prostatic hypertrophy)**    I mention this disorder possibly to save you from prostate surgery.

The prostate grows with age and can cause obstruction to urinary flow, incomplete emptying of the bladder, and urine infections. (When urine remains in the bladder, the few bacteria in it multiply.)

Until recently this problem was thought to be caused by a mechanical obstruction. It has been shown, however, that nerves that control sphincter muscles in the urethra may be overactive. If the nerve activity is decreased (using a medication such as Minipress), the spasm can often improve and the rate of urinary flow will increase. In particular, urine retention in the bladder may cease, and as a result so will infections.

I have had patients use this treatment successfully for years. Even if it can delay prostate surgery for a time, it is worthwhile to try. The drugs are reasonably well tolerated, especially by the elderly men in whom this condition tends to occur.

If your doctor does not mention this treatment, bring it up. It does not seem to be well known yet. Max B, an older patient from a Midwestern city, consults me when his doctors do not help or he does not like what they say. After being advised to have prostate surgery "by two of the biggest urologists in town," he was amazed when his symptoms disappeared when I prescribed Minipress. "Why didn't they prescribe this for me?" he asked.

**6. Cancer of the Prostate**     Prostate cancer is one of the big killers and its frequency is far greater than most people suppose. Its likelihood increases with age. (Most men by the time they reach the age of eighty will have at least a few cancer cells in their prostate.)

Prostate cancer can often be detected during a routine physical by having the physician palpate the prostate. If he feels a hard nodule in the prostate, further investigation is most certainly warranted.

Only twenty years ago a diagnosis of cancer of the prostate was likely to be a death sentence. Since then, however, remarkable advances have taken place that may allow the sufferer to live a relatively normal life, depending on the stage of the cancer when first detected.

An annual prostate examination is your best weapon against this problem. Since not all cancers can be felt, some doctors also recommend a blood test, serum prostate specific antigen. If the level is elevated, it suggests that cancer may be present in the prostate.

If either of these tests is abnormal, a prostate ultrasound can be ordered. Ultrasounds are too expensive to be used routinely in prostate cancer screening but can help your doctor confirm a diagnosis if other tests suggest its use. Screening for prostate cancer in males over the age of fifty-five should be performed routinely, as should breast cancer screening (mammogram) and uterine cervical cancer screening (Pap smear) for women.

# 8
## Chest Pain

When we have chest pain, we immediately worry that it's a heart attack. Prudently, most of us will go to an emergency room or doctor to have the pain diagnosed and treated.

Nevertheless, most chest pain is not caused by a heart condition. Some may be caused by acidity or by other intestinal conditions, as we saw in Chapter 6. Much chest pain is caused by muscle or bone problems, or inflammation or blood clots in the lungs could be involved.

The trouble is that once you've seen your doctor about your chest pain and he's eliminated your heart as a problem, he may simply lose interest. Somehow the implication is that if your heart and associated structures are normal, your condition is not serious and hence you needn't worry about it. Unfortunately, this still leaves you with the pain.

What do you do?

In this chapter we look at chest pain that is not associated with any heart or lung problems. We will see some of the things that cause it and look at some treatments you can ask your doctor about.

But don't self-diagnose chest pain! If you have chest pain, you should immediately be evaluated by your doctor for a heart or lung problem. Only after you are certain you do not have a heart condition, consider the following possibilities.

### ESOPHAGEAL PAIN

The esophagus is the tube that connects the throat to the stomach. Pain in the esophagus is one of the two main causes of chest pain not associated with the heart or lungs.

Esophageal pain itself can come from two sources. One is

a disorder in which stomach acids backwash and burn the esophagus, causing the sensation of chest pain. This ailment (called gastroesophageal reflux) was discussed in Chapter 6.

The other cause involves spasm of the esophageal muscles (esophageal motility disorder) and resultant pain.

**DIAGNOSING ESOPHAGEAL PAIN**  If you have chest pain and your doctor doesn't think it has anything to do with your cardiac system, he can check to find out if it has something to do with your esophagus by asking you to take an antacid to see if this helps. If it does, it may indicate a stomach problem.

However, an antacid may not help if you are having heartburn and will not help in other esophageal disorders. An upper GI X-ray or esophagoscopy may not give a clear-cut diagnosis either.

One test that many doctors rarely perform gives good answers to this question and should be used more often. It involves the injection of a drug called edrophonium (Tensilon).

Tensilon is used primarily to diagnose a muscle-weakness disorder called myasthenia gravis and has some limited use in heart-rhythm problems. Its benefit here, however, is that when injected it can provoke chest pain in people with esophageal disorders. In other words, if your doctor injects you with this drug and you get chest pain, it strongly suggests that your problem is located in the esophagus.

Unfortunately, this test does not distinguish between problems caused by reflux, those caused by movement of food, and those caused by spasm of the esophagus. Nevertheless, just identifying that the problem is in the esophagus is a good start.

Once your doctor knows the problem is in the esophagus, he can try you on an anti-acid-backwash regimen. Usually this treatment will include agents to decrease stomach acidity or to empty your stomach more rapidly. He or she may suggest elevating the head of your bed while you sleep.

**DIAGNOSTIC TECHNIQUES AND THEIR DRAW-BACKS**  While a Tensilon test is relatively simple and fairly accurate, some doctors want to be more precise. They want to know exactly what the problem is. The difficulty is that diagnosing esophageal pain caused by spasm (a motility disorder) is very hard, to do. There are no easily discovered clear-cut answers, although there are a wide variety of tests. Some of these tests may be suggested for you. You would be wise to consider seriously whether you want to have them, since their results may be of questionable value.

For example, some doctors actually suggest that a patient walk around for a day with a tube in his nose and down his throat to record esophageal pressure. The purpose of this procedure is to see if there is increased pain when there is increased pressure (spasm).

Others may want to inflate a balloon in the esophagus to see whether there will be pain when it is distended. Of course there will, but the question they will ask is whether or not this pain occurs with less distension than for normal people. The problem is that no one knows what is the maximum distension before pain should occur.

If your doctor recommends these tests, ask him what he hopes to learn from them. The results may not warrant the effort.

**TREATMENTS OF QUESTIONABLE VALUE** In addition to possibly unwarranted diagnostic tests, some treatments are of dubious utility for motility disorders of the esophagus. For example, some doctors suggest treating spasms of the esophagus with calcium channel blockers, which reduce spasm. However, double-blind studies have not shown that they reduce pain. Since there are so few therapeutic choices, these drugs may nevertheless be prescribed.

Other doctors may believe it worthwhile to try a medication called octreotide (Sandostatin), which affects the nerves controlling gut motility. I have not seen anything in the medical literature about the benefits of this use, however. Sandostatin could actually make your symptoms worse, but your doctor may feel it is worth trying in a difficult situation.

Still other doctors may try using a drug called leuprolide acetate (Lupron). This medication will supposedly stop any manifestation of irritable gut, in an appropriate dosage. But it will also put women into artificial menopause.

These are some of the possible treatments for esophageal spasm. The problem is that they do not often result in any relief of symptoms and can cause adverse reactions.

Unfortunately, I have no easy answers either.

Probably the best, albeit imperfect, way to treat esophageal pains as of now is to try to modify whatever makes the esophagus irritable. If food passage is the problem, softer food and smaller pieces may help. Antireflux measures can be helpful if spasm is caused by acid backwash from the stomach.

My suggestion, however, is that if you have an esophageal motility disorder, be aware that there is no simple answer. If your doctor suggests one of the tests or remedies we've discussed here, it may help you, but do not expect it to be a panacea. You may have a malady that has no definite treatment at the present time. Psychiatric consultation is sometimes recommended since esophageal motility disorders are seen more often in anxious people.

## MUSCLE AND BONE (MUSCULOSKELETAL) CHEST PAIN

The most commonly overlooked diagnosis in the patient with chest pain other than heart problem or a problem with the esophagus is musculoskeletal. Some doctors check for heart problems and then, when there are none, may push on the junction of the ribs and the breastbone to see whether that maneuver reproduces the chest pain. If it does they may nod and prescribe anti-inflammatory drugs to treat what they think is inflammation of the joints between the ribs and the breastbone. Unfortunately, many physicians do little more than that, and the anti-inflammatory drugs may only have a transient benefit if they have any at all.

### DIAGNOSING MUSCULOSKELETAL CHEST PAIN

The muscles that most commonly cause chest pain that could be mistaken for angina are those over the front of the chest and ribs (pectoralis major and minor). You may even be able to diagnose this problem yourself by feeling for trigger points (see Chapter 1) on your own. Grab your chest muscles between the thumb and forefinger and, starting at your armpit, squeeze them all the way down your chest.

Do this procedure while sitting with your arm out at a ninety-degree angle. If you squeeze a trigger point, it should reproduce the pain at the location as well as elsewhere in your chest and perhaps even down your arm, if that symptom also occurs. This test may even produce momentary numbness down your arm.

**WHAT CAUSES THIS TYPE OF PAIN?** These trigger points can be caused by any activity that would involve your arms coming together in front of you, like using hedge clippers. They can also be caused by poor posture. If you stand with a slump, you eventually cause the muscles to shorten, and shortened muscles are more apt to spasm and develop trigger points. There is even a spot in the muscle on the lower right side (the lower pectoralis major) that can cause irregular or rapid heartbeats.

**TREATMENT** I described the treatment for trigger points in detail in Chapter 1. Briefly, it involves injecting the trigger points with a mild salt solution (normal saline) or spraying the muscles with a coolant and then stretching them. Long-term treatment involves improving your posture. A simple exercise may also help. Stand in an open doorway and rest your forearms on the sides of the doorframe. Then lean forward. This action will stretch your pectoral muscles, and doing it repeatedly may help eliminate trigger points.

**MUSCULOSKELETAL CHEST PAIN WITH HEART TROUBLE** Real problems arise if you have both heart trouble and muscle/bone problems. You may have anginal chest pain or even a heart attack and may also have trigger points in your pectoral muscles. The great danger is that your doctor might treat the trigger points and thus eliminate most of the pain. This could lull him into a false sense of security and cause him to miss your heart problem. (A thorough doctor should be aware that with heart problems some deep pressure-type pain might remain under the breastbone and a little lower in the region of the stomach even after the trigger points are eliminated.)

I never give trigger-point injections into chest muscles unless I am certain that the patient has no heart disease. The very act of injection releases a muscle enzyme (CPK) that is measured in a blood test to diagnose heart attacks. Thus the injection could cause the diagnosis of a heart condition by mistake.

## CHEST WALL PAIN

Numerous muscles and bones in the chest wall can cause pain. Chest-wall pain usually begins abruptly, is sharp and stabbing, and can last a long time or resolve in a moment. It is made worse by movement. If you touch your chest it will usually be tender, particularly at the junctions of the ribs with the breastbone (usually the second through the fifth rib), a condition technically called costochondritis.

One way you can determine if costochondritis is your problem is to stretch these areas. Since they are joints and not muscles, stretching will make the pain worse.

To stretch these joints, try the "crowing rooster" maneuver. Stretch your arms out at your sides and have someone pull them backward. If you have costochondritis, this movement should make your pain worse. If not, the pain could be coming from the sternalis muscle, which is alongside the breastbone and has no known function.

Both pains can be relieved by injection of an appropriate solution into the tender areas.

## ARTHRITIS

Sometimes doctors miss the fact that arthritis can cause chest pain, even when the chest is not involved directly.

People who have arthritis in the upper part of the spine, the neck and the upper chest often have arthritis of the facet joints between the vertebrae (the bones of the spine). This condition may manifest itself as chest pain and can be quite severe, unrelenting, and difficult to treat.

If you have chest pain caused by facet arthritis, ask your doctor about neck exercises, which are sometimes helpful. Another remedy may be nonsteroidal anti-inflammatory drugs such as ibuprofen (Advil, Motrin).

The pain also may be helped by having your doctor inject cortisone around the spinal cord, a procedure called epidural steroid injection that is often quite effective and can be used from neck down to tailbone. Epidural steroid injection is a generally safe procedure and is underutilized in areas other than the lower back. It is helpful in disc disease too, if the disc (the cushion between the vertebrae) has not slipped (herniated) too far.

If you have neck pain and stiffness accompanying your chest pain, you may have "pseudoangina," caused by compression of the spinal cord from spinal arthritis in the neck. Many patients with pseudoangina see one or two heart specialists before the diagnosis is made. Treatment begins with a cervical collar, anti-inflammatory drugs, and traction.

## SHINGLES AND CHEST PAIN

Another type of chest pain that is fairly preventable is caused by shingles (herpes zoster).

Herpes zoster is produced by the same virus that causes chickenpox. The virus remains dormant in the body after the initial infection. Then, many years afterward, for reasons not well understood it travels from the spinal cord along a single nerve, usually between the ribs. For the first few days there will be tingling and pain in the chest, then a rash that looks like chickenpox will spread in a line along the nerve. Some sufferers describe the pain as an "electric lightning bolt."

**TREATMENT FOR SHINGLES** A problem may arise if you see your doctor with herpes zoster pain before the rash develops. He or she may not recognize the symptoms and, consequently, may not start treatment immediately. A delay in treatment may result in a poor outcome. Be sure to ask about shingles if your symptoms are anything similar to those described above.

The usual therapy involves high doses of the medication acyclovir (Zovirax), usually four times as much as your doctor would use to treat a cold sore (herpes simplex). Another drug, an H-2 blocker, is sometimes used as well. Some physicians also prescribe cortisone (or cortisone alone), but I don't feel this is the treatment of choice.

Shingles usually resolves rapidly if treated appropriately and promptly.

If you believe you have shingles, don't delay in seeing your doctor. The longer shingles last, the more apt they are to damage the involved nerve all the way back to where it comes out of the spinal cord. Ten percent of patients with herpes zoster develop postherpetic neuralgia, a severe, burning, numbing pain along the course of the nerve that is difficult to treat.

**IF IT DOESN'T GO AWAY**   Sometimes shingles won't go away quickly. If you have ever seen anyone with this disorder in a chronic state, you will appreciate how painful it can be. What's worse, postherpetic neuralgia can last months and months.

Your doctor should use additional medications for postherpetic neuralgia. The best treatment is probably a medication called capsaicin (Zostrix) in cream form. It affects a chemical produced by the nerve that helps to transmit pain. Zostrix has also been used successfully in nerve pain caused by diabetes. Your doctor may also want to give you antidepressants and other drugs such as haloperidol (Haldol) to decrease the pain of postherpetic neuralgia.

A technique called transcutaneous electrical nerve stimulation (TENS) is also effective. It uses skin-patch electrodes to send electrical signals along larger nerves into the spinal cord to attempt to block pain impulses that travel along smaller nerves. A variety of procedures has been used to cut or destroy the nerves that mediate the pain of postherpetic neuralgia. None is uniformly effective and I will recommend them only in the most severe cases. The disorder is agonizing for the patient and particularly frustrating for the physician who is trying to help.

# 9
=

# Headaches

If you occasionally get a headache, take an aspirin, and find that the headache quickly goes away, you should consider yourself fortunate. For many people, a simple headache that can be cured by an aspirin is something they wish they could have. Instead, they have severe chronic headaches that may disable them for long periods of time.

Headaches have many causes, some of which your doctor may miss. That's most unfortunate, since there are many exciting new headache treatments just gaining medical acceptance.

My object here in writing about headaches is therefore to highlight certain aspects of headache diagnosis and treatment that I find some other physicians frequently overlook. My purpose is to tell you about areas of headache medicine in which your doctor may not have been trained so you can discuss a diagnosis or treatment which he or she did not consider.

## A HEADACHE PROBLEM

As the medical director of a pain and stress management center I frequently see patients with intractable headaches. Often, by the time they reach me these people have been to several doctors and have received several diagnoses, one or more of which may be wrong.

For example, when Madeline came to me she was having one to two headaches a week. She had been to doctors for several years; the diagnoses had been only partial and vague. Over the course of time she had been told she had three different types of headaches. One was a cluster headache.

**CLUSTER HEADACHE**   Madeline was told a cluster headache was a form of a migraine. She would wake up from a sound sleep with a blinding pain. The pain would diminish but could last for weeks and be accompanied by mild nausea. She would get this type of headache only rarely.

I examined her and discovered that she actually did not have any of the symptoms of cluster headaches. Cluster headaches occur primarily in men, usually last a fairly short time, and are associated with watering of the eye and nasal discharge on the side of the pain, which is quite severe. They are called cluster headaches because they occur in bunches, then may disappear for varying periods of time. Occurrence is usually random, but sometimes they are seasonal. Although it did not help her problem, she was relieved to hear that cluster headaches were not part of it.

**SINUS HEADACHES**   Madeline had also been told she had sinus headaches. She felt severe pressure behind her eyebrows. She said ''When it comes, it feels like my face is going to explode.'' She associated these headaches with low barometric pressure or fog. They occurred three or four times a year and lasted a few minutes to a day. A nasal decongestant spray accompanied by moist heat made her feel better and often relieved the headache. She did appear to have sinus headaches.

**TENSION-TYPE, OR STRESS HEADACHES**   Finally, several doctors had told Madeline that her headaches were caused by stress; therefore she had stress headaches, which she experienced as pressure in her temples and at the base of her neck.

These particular headaches came several times a week and consequently were her primary complaint. They caused her to miss work or to work ineffectively. While I told her that the term *stress headache* was misleading, stress certainly did play a role in these headaches. (They are called tension-type headaches in medical parlance.)

The reason that Madeline came to see me was that her previous doctors had not been able to give her much relief from these various kinds of headaches other than to prescribe pain medications and to encourage her to relax.

''It's the stress headaches that really bother me,'' she said. ''Because they're always there. I've lost two jobs because of them and I'm in trouble right now at my present job. Only nobody seems to be able to do anything about them!''

**NOT COOKBOOK HEADACHES** The problem, of course, was that Madeline's headaches did not fit into the usual description of headaches doctors are familiar with. In truth, perhaps only 5 to 10 percent of her headaches fit the medical cookbook. What bothered her the most were the other 90 percent, those that had been given the wastebasket term *stress headaches*. The doctors she had seen did not have a quick and easy remedy for them—or any effective treatment at all.

This chapter, then, looks into those headaches that may have been lumped under the heading *stress*. Our goal is to find solutions to headache problems that your doctor overlooked. In doing this we will also consider some of the standard headaches, including those due to sinus congestion and migraines, with which most doctors are familiar and for which treatment is standardized but not always prescribed effectively.

## STRESS HEADACHES

As noted, most of the headaches in this gray area are called muscle-contraction headaches or tension-type headaches. They may be mild but can occur on a daily or continuous basis. They can be so severe that you must go to bed. They have a variety of causes.

This group of vaguely defined headaches is far and away the most common kind I see—and probably the kind most people suffer from. Perhaps the headache you may be feeling is one of these.

**NOT RELATED TO MUSCLE TENSION** First, understand that this most common form of headache is misnamed. It is usually not related to tension or to muscle contraction at all. Rather, they are most frequently caused by trigger points in certain muscles in the head, neck, and upper back (see Chapter 1).

Unfortunately, many doctors even today are completely unfamiliar with trigger points as they relate to headaches. I have read hundreds of articles on headaches and rarely see trigger points even mentioned. Most physicians have not been trained to examine patients for trigger points, let alone to eliminate them. They consequently overlook them in their diagnostic procedures.

**TRIGGER POINTS IN STRESS HEADACHES**   A trigger point is a tender area in a muscle that can cause local pain and—more important here—can also refer pain to a distant site. We do not understand very well how trigger points are formed or what they really are. However, once you know about them, locating them is usually quite easy. When I press on a trigger point with my finger, it is tender, the patient usually winces and contracts the muscle, and the process may cause referred pain at a site quite distant from the location of the trigger point.

Very often when a person complains about one of these "other" headaches, what he or she really has are trigger points referring pain to the head.

**INDICATIONS OF TRIGGER-POINT HEADACHES**
While a physician who has been trained to locate trigger points can most easily find them, you can locate some of them yourself. If you have headaches, there may be two or three trigger points on the front edge of the muscle on top of your shoulders that contracts when you shrug your shoulders (the trapezius). The trapezius trigger point nearest your neck is the most common culprit and can cause pain to radiate up the neck, along the side of the head, and to a spot that feels like it is right behind the eye. (One of the most common complaints of headache sufferers is pain that seems to be located right behind the eye.)

Another trigger point that causes neck pain is in the muscle in the shoulder called the levator scapulae. This trigger point takes some training to find. It attaches to the shoulder blade, sometimes called the wing bone, more properly termed the scapula. The muscle elevates this bone when the shoulders are shrugged. It is almost always associated with trigger points in the trapezius.

Many tense people frequently contract these muscles without being aware of doing so. This straining may cause the trigger points to develop over time. These trigger points are also common in occupations that require a seated employee to bend over. I see them frequently in secretaries, manicurists, and dental hygienists. Madeline was a secretary.)

**SELF-EXAM** To feel these trigger points yourself, wet your shoulders with water or moisturizing cream and exert steady pressure as you move your fingers from the side of your neck along the top of your shoulder. Move your fingers along until you find a small pea-sized nodule that is painful to the touch. You've found your first trigger point. Press it and you may feel pain where you press as well as the headache pain you couldn't quite identify before.

You can find other trigger points in a similar fashion, but nodules will not be present in most locations.

## CLENCHED- OR GRINDING-TEETH HEADACHES

While trigger points in the shoulders and neck are the most common cause of headaches I see, the second most common kind of headache in my patients is related to grinding and clenching of the teeth, or bruxism. People grind their teeth while awake and frequently while asleep. Chewing gum can worsen this condition. As with the muscles of the neck and shoulders, trigger points in the muscles of the jaw may eventually develop. Most people who grind or clench their teeth at night are not aware that they do it. The first indication may be a comment by your dentist that your teeth are wearing down rapidly or developing small fractures.

**SELF-EXAM** The primary chewing muscle is called the masseter. You can feel the masseter if you place your index finger about an inch in front of your earlobe and then open and close your mouth. Be gentle as you do this; if you have trigger points in your masseter, this maneuver may cause pain.

Another way to see if you have trigger points in your masseter is to gently squeeze the muscle with your thumb and forefinger. With your thumb on the outside of your face and your forefinger inside your mouth, sequentially squeeze your masseter from your cheekbone down to your lower jaw.

The masseter can contain several sets of trigger points. If

you have more than one set, you will not feel entirely well until all sets are inactivated.

**RELATED EAR PAIN**    Masseter trigger points are also a frequent cause of ear pain when no other cause can be found. Other trigger points associated with the masseter are frequently found in the muscle located on your temple just above your ear (the temporalis). You should be able to feel them fairly easily by moving your finger up from your ear. Look for these associated trigger points if you find them in the masseter itself. If you have a masseter spasm you will not be able to open your mouth widely enough to insert the knuckles of three fingers.

## NOT TEMPOROMANDIBULAR SYNDROME

I'm not writing here about the temporomandibular joint syndrome or TMJ syndrome that many people are concerned about. TMJ syndrome refers to an actual malfunction of the joint where the jawbone fits into the head. Because of the need for a more encompassing term, the various disorders have recently been renamed the temporomandibular pain and dysfunction syndrome (TMPDS), to include all causes. TMPDS may sometimes be part of the fibromyalgia syndrome discussed in Chapter 1.

There is almost never anything wrong with the joint itself unless there has been a severe injury to it or you have joint disease such as rheumatoid arthritis. Unfortunately, some doctors are inclined to diagnose it to please their patients or because they cannot find another cause. I have personally seen several teeth-grinding-headache patients who have been incorrectly advised by the doctors that they have TMJ syndrome and that they should have surgery to correct it.

If your doctor suggests surgery, it should only be as a last resort after trying other treatments. I have never treated a patient with this problem where surgery was required. (Some of my patients, however, previously had surgery and reported that it did help them.)

Remember, the headache problem may more likely be caused by teeth-grinding or clenching, which in turn causes trigger points, than by TMJ syndrome. Before you rush off to have surgery on your joints, seriously investigate the possibility that the real problem may be elsewhere.

## SINUS AND TOOTH PROBLEMS AS HEADACHE CAUSES

People who have headaches that commonly occur when they wake up in the morning may have sinus headaches. These headaches commonly decrease when standing but recur as the day goes on. Many patients who have pain in their teeth and may have had numerous root canals and other dental procedures actually have dental pain that is felt as a headache. You may want to ask your dentist if your teeth could be the cause of your headache. We discuss sinuses in Chapter 11.

Many patients who feel pain in their teeth actually have myofascial pain caused by temporomandibular pain and dysfunction syndrome. There often will be trigger points in the masseter and the temporalis muscles that can be easily felt, and thermography (a technique that measures and displays temperature in the body as areas of different colors) will have characteristic findings of TMPDS.

## TRIGEMINAL NEURALGIA

Trigeminal neuralgia or tic douloureux, a disorder of the nerve that supplies sensation to the face, may cause headaches. Patients with trigeminal neuralgia usually have sudden stabbing pain that is very severe in the areas where the trigeminal nerve is found. Dental pain may sometimes be confused with trigeminal neuralgia, but I have been struck with how often trigeminal neuralgia is misdiagnosed.

Several years ago I participated in a double-blind experiment for a possible new treatment for trigeminal neuralgia. I had to screen the patients to make sure they actually met the criteria for the diagnosis. I saw quite a few patients and was surprised at how many actually had TMPDS—more than half of them. (I am sure I had a biased sample, because patients with trigeminal neuralgia who were diagnosed and treated properly probably would not have volunteered for the experiment.)

### TREATING OTHER HEADACHES

Your doctor can treat your trigger-point or tooth-grinding headache quite well, once a correct diagnosis is made. For example, if the problem is trigger points, stretching the muscle after injections of a saline solution (see Chapter 1) work very well.

In addition, for trigger points that produce headaches the following treatments may be helpful and you may want to bring them up with your doctor.

The trigger points can be stimulated with ultrasound or electrically with an Acuscope, an instrument that is applied to the acupuncture points.

The individual muscle can be stretched to try to break up the local area of spasm. As the muscle is stretched, your doctor or physical therapist may use a cold spray (called Fluorimethane) directed at a thirty-degree angle along the muscle from the trigger point to the area of referred pain to help stretch it.

The trigger points causing headaches can be massaged. Vibration and pulsating minor electric shocks are helpful. Transcutaneous electrical nerve stimulation (TENS) may help block nerve transmission of pain into the spinal cord.

It is not necessary to inject your trigger points with a cortisone derivative. Cortison should only be injected into areas of inflammation. Trigger points are not inflamed structures.

**MADELINE'S RESPONSE TO TREATMENT**   A good result from a trigger-point injection should be the rapid disappearance of the trigger point and its associated headache. This is what happened to Madeline, who had trigger points in her neck and shoulders. I injected eight of them and within a few minutes, to her amazement, her headache was gone. With the appropriate stretching exercises it did not return.

**GETTING AT ROOT CAUSES**   This result highlights the fact that while treatment can produce dramatic results, the headache itself will often recur unless the true causes are corrected. This task is best accomplished by tackling the problem on several fronts at once, including:

Physical therapy
Psychotherapy
Biofeedback
Stress management
Therapeutic exercise

These may produce the kind of long-term "cure" you are really looking for.

I try to avoid frequent use of certain drugs sometimes prescribed for headaches such as ergotamine, narcotics, or phenobarbital (as in Fiorinal) because patients can have rebound headaches when they wear off, causing them to use these drugs more frequently, thus perpetuating the headache.

**Biofeedback**   Biofeedback has gotten a kind of pop celebrity because of which many people think of it as being hooked up to a machine and being asked to try to raise and lower blood pressure. Modern biofeedback differs greatly from this model. The technique is a very sophisticated discipline involving the monitoring of multiple physiologic parameters by a trained specialist who is also an expert in stress reduction. The basis of biofeedback is that a person can learn voluntarily to control bodily functions he may have been unaware of or that were previously thought to be involuntary if he is given continuous feedback about their measurement. If you want to try biofeedback, be sure that your doctor or the practitioner he or she recommends is specially trained in stress reduction as well. Otherwise you may get poor results, not because of the failure of biofeedback but because of the lack of expertise of the therapist.

**OTHER TREATMENTS**   Sometimes a headache seems intractable and the techniques suggested above do not work. Your doctor may then want to prescribe medications. If beta blockers such as propanolol (Inderal) and tricyclic antidepressants such as amitriptylene (Elavil) are ineffective, your doctor may then want to consider whether your headache is due to overactivity of the sympathetic nervous system, which uses chemicals related to adrenalin to transmit impulses. Two drugs that block the action of these chemicals you can discuss with your physician are prazosin (Minipress), which is also used for hypertension, and prostatodynia or clonidine (Catapres), also used for high blood pressure and for drug withdrawal. Clonidine is a pain reliever in its own right, a fact that I discovered several years ago and which has been confirmed by others since.

A more dramatic and possibly better way to decrease sympathetic nerve activity is to receive a sympathetic nerve block. This can be done by injecting a local anesthetic into the bundle (ganglion) of sympathetic nerves that go to the head and face.

Sometimes this sympathetic nerve block will relieve the pain dramatically. If it does, your doctor can repeat the block as needed and the pain relief may last longer each time it is done.

## MIGRAINES

Having discussed some of the ''other'' headaches, which are the bulk of those experienced, let's now concentrate on migraines. Only 10 to 15 percent of the population have migraines but many people think they have them since severe headaches are commonly called migraines.

In recent years the concept of migraine headaches has been expanded to overlap with other types of headaches, perhaps because classical migraine, in which constriction and expansion of the arteries in the brain are involved, comprises only 15 to 20 percent of those with migraines. Other types of headaches include ''common'' migraine, which lasts longer and does not generally have artery constriction associated with it, and tension-type headaches. There are also ''mixed'' headaches, a combination of tension-type and migraine. It may be worthwhile for your doctor to try treating all of them with similar agents.

Migraines occur on one side of the head only, and have associated symptoms:

Sensitivity to light
Nausea or vomiting
Auras, often scintillating blind spots or scotoma (seen in classical migraine only)

Migraines are easily recognized by doctors. If you suffer from them, your doctor should be able to make the diagnosis and should also be able to prescribe treatment that is usually effective. However, sometimes the headache isn't relieved. When your doctor can't help you with your migraine, first be sure that the diagnosis is correct. There are a number of disorders causing headache with which migraines can be confused, including:

Drugs or drug withdrawal
Trigeminal neuralgia
Brain tumor or aneurysm
Brain hemorrhage
Eyestrain
Sinusitis
Allergy problems
Infections or metabolic disorders

Be sure that your doctor has examined you for and eliminated all of these. Once he has, you might want to discuss with him some of the treatments outlined below. First, however, it's helpful to understand what happens when you have a migraine.

**UNDERSTANDING MIGRAINE** The cause of migraine is still unclear. There are several theories. One of the most popular is the "carotid shunt" theory. The carotid artery carries blood to the brain. The blood is metabolized by the brain and then removed by veins. The muscles of the shunt arteries are regulated by serotonin. Although it is not completely understood why it happens, when a migraine occurs the blood bypasses the metabolic area and goes directly from artery to vein by opening of a shunt, which also increases blood flow. The closing of this shunt and the opening of the area of the brain that was excluded through the use of sumatriptan and other agents that affect serotonin, should relieve the headache.

**TREATING MIGRAINES** Your doctor may use a variety of medications to treat your migraine. These include something as simple as aspirin in low doses. The antidepressant Prozac, which can actually cause migraines, can help in controlling them. Beta blockers and tricyclic antidepressants are commonly used. Calcium channel blockers, which prevent artery spasm, are also very useful agents. As a result of severe artery constriction, patients with migraines have had strokes (death of nerve cells caused by lack of blood supply).

**Migraines and Menstruation**   Some migraine headaches occur with menstruation and can probably be related to an increased amount of chemicals (prostaglandins) in the blood. The lining of the uterus is rich in these substances and is expelled each month in the menstrual contents and built up anew. As the prostaglandin-rich uterine lining is expelled, these chemicals circulate in the bloodstream and perhaps cause migraines.

Your doctor may use medications that block the formation of prostaglandins called nonsteroidal anti-inflammatory drugs, such as ibuprofen (Advil, Motrin), which is available over the counter. They are also the medications of choice for menstrual cramps.

**Other Treatments**   There are several other kinds of anti-migraine treatments. Two that are not well known are the medications captopril (Capoten) and enalapril (Vasotec), both used to treat high blood pressure and heart failure. These can sometimes prevent headaches when taken regularly. You may want to discuss using these drugs with your doctor if yours is a case that has not responded to other treatments.

# 10

## Asthma

Asthmatic patients once had to rely more on willpower than anything else in their attempts to lead a normal life. There was relatively little that medicine could offer them.

Fortunately, that has changed. In the last ten years or so, therapy has become quite scientific. Today there are many different medications and precise ways of determining which to give. Now asthma can almost always be controlled so that a patient can lead a relatively normal life.

I am therefore continually amazed at the number of asthmatic patients who come to my office inadequately treated. Some physicians clearly still know very little about the advances that have been made.

This chapter explains the nature of asthma and discusses current treatment. If you find your doctor is not helping your asthmatic condition, you may want to read the following pages carefully, then discuss some of the suggested therapies.

### WHAT IS ASTHMA?

An asthmatic has an airway that overreacts to various stimuli—smoke, pollens, and the like. The airway is composed of the windpipe (trachea) and the tubes that stem from it (the bronchi) leading into the lungs. In asthmatics the airway is described as being twitchy, which means that, because of its hyper-reactive nature, it constricts inappropriately. When the airway constricts there is a tightening of the muscles around the bronchi, inflammation and swelling of the lining of the bronchi, and secretion of mucus and other liquids by cells that live in the lining. When the twitchy bronchial tubes narrow or constrict too much, the result is coughing and wheezing.

Asthma therapy is aimed at altering these responses.

## WHAT CAUSES ASTHMA?

We do not know the cause of asthma. There may, in fact, be several causes which produce a similar result. Wheezing asthma in children is likely to be related to allergy, perhaps to substances in the air such as pollen. It is rarely related to foods. Some psychologists have noted that asthmatic children are found more often in dysfunctional families, indicating that there may be an emotional component in some cases of childhood asthma.

It is when asthma begins in adult life that we know very little about what causes it; we do know that it is almost never related to allergy, and giving allergy shots to decrease airway reactivity is used in adults only as a last resort. However, whether allergy is a factor or not, if you have asthma, you should prepare a dust-free bedroom, since dust mites and other fine particles can make the airway twitch during sleep and cause difficult breathing.

## TREATING ASTHMA

The symptoms of asthma are produced by either an excess or a deficiency of certain chemicals in the bronchi. Since we do not know how to treat the cause, we treat the symptoms by increasing or decreasing the concentrations of some of these chemicals.

The symptoms are also caused by certain kinds of cells that secrete specific chemicals, particularly ones that cause inflammation. We try to decrease the movement of these cells into the airway in the second (late) phase of the asthmatic response.

**INHALATION TREATMENT**    A cardinal principle of treating all disease is to achieve the maximum benefit with the fewest adverse effects or risks. This objective can often be accomplished in asthma by giving a drug so that it only goes to the area where it is needed and is not absorbed into the rest of the body. Asthmatics can do this by inhaling their medications into their bronchi through the mouth. Avoid systemic medications, usually taken in pill form, unless inhalers cannot control the symptoms.

Four drugs can be delivered to the bronchial lining by inhalation. Discuss these with your physician to see if one or more would be useful for you.

1. Albuterol (Proventil, Ventolin), metaproterenol (Alupent) or terbutaline (Brethaire)—beta-2 receptor-stimulating drugs. These act to relax the tight muscles around the bronchi and are usually prescribed first.
2. Corticosteroids, beclomethasone (Vanceril, Beclovent) or triamcinolone (Azmacort). These drugs allow the bronchodilating chemicals to be more effective, decrease the tendency of bronchial cells that secrete inflammatory chemicals to react to stimuli, and block the production of powerful constricting chemicals (leukotrienes).
3. Cromolyn (Intal). This drug affects calcium metabolism in some bronchial cells so they do not secrete chemicals that inflame and constrict the bronchi and attract other inflammatory cells. It is the safest asthma drug and is useful in treating children.
4. Atropine and ipratopium bromide (Atrovent). These medications block a chemical, acetylcholine, that causes the bronchi to constrict and secrete fluid.

## PUSHING INHALANT THERAPY

The tendency of many physicians is to start systemic medication as soon as it appears that the inhaled drugs described above are not working by themselves. This may not be necessary. Making sure inhalers are used properly and in the right sequence, or increasing the dosage of the drugs they dispense may change a nonresponder into a responder.

I usually do not start systemic medication until I have my patients use all four inhalers in combination, beginning with the beta stimulator. Using it first expands or dilates the bronchi so that the other inhaled drugs can penetrate further.

Inhalers are prescribed to deliver medication that would normally be used systemically, like cortisone drugs. (These agents, if taken systemically, produce a tendency to become fat in the face and trunk, thin the bones, and have other adverse side effects—including increased susceptibility to infection.)

The inhaled corticosteroids usually accomplish this goal of

local treatment. However, the dosage in which they are normally prescribed—two puffs four times a day, for a total of eight—may be inadequate. There is evidence that they can be given more often, as many as sixteen or thirty-two times a day, with minimal systemic effects. (In Canada, high-dose corticosteroid inhalers are available so that patients do not have to take so many inhalations.)

This change is the easiest single modification I can make in the treatment regimen of an asthmatic patient. Increased frequency of dosage can markedly improve a condition and may enable the asthmatic to stop or avoid taking corticosteroids systemically.

Inhaled corticosteroids may also prevent you from developing tolerance to the effects of inhaled beta-2 receptor-stimulating drugs, although some studies show that tolerance may not occur anyway.

Usually, beta-2 inhalers should be used regularly. Increased difficulty with breathing is a clue that the dosage of the steroid inhaler should be increased by the physician.

If fluid secretion is a prominent symptom, I use ipratropium bromide (Atrovent). This agent usually dries up secretions and may confer added benefit when used with a beta stimulator.

It's not just that four different inhalers can be used. How, in what order, and in what dose they are used counts most. Discuss this aspect of treatment in detail with your physician if you are not responding well and he or she wants you to use systemic drugs.

## JUDGING HOW WELL YOU ARE DOING

Response to therapy should not be assessed only by how well you feel. You may be feeling all right, but actually still be in trouble. For example, the normal airway diameter can be reduced by 50 percent without causing wheezing or shortness of breath when you are not exerting yourself. You might stop using your inhalers too soon if you judge your condition only by how well you feel.

Rather, a scientific measurement should be made. Since asthma characteristically reduces the volume of forcibly exhaled air, we measure this capacity to exhale by a technique, called spirometry, that records and graphs exhaled airflow. If you are asthmatic, you have probably had (or should have had) spirometry to assess the adequacy of your therapy. Some asthmatics do spirometry at home and adjust their medication accordingly.

## SYSTEMIC TREATMENT

Sometimes inhalers are simply not sufficient to control symptoms. The next drug prescribed is usually some form of theophylline.

**THEOPHYLLINE** Theophylline may act primarily by blocking a chemical called adenosine, which is also blocked by caffeine. Adenosine has a somewhat sedating effect, and by blocking it in the brain with theophylline makes some people nervous. However, the medication may also have an anti-inflammatory effect that may be more important.

Unfortunately, theophylline is not effective when inhaled. It is taken by mouth in the form of pills or capsules.

**Problems with Theophylline** Some of the problems with theophylline are nausea, vomiting, nervousness, and heart palpitations. It may also interfere with learning and concentration. This was caused, in part, by our belief that high doses were needed. We used to think that, to be effective, theophylline must reach a certain level in the blood. If the level was too low, it would not work as a bronchodilator, and if too high, adverse effects would commonly ensue. Monitoring of theo-phylline levels by blood tests was an essential aspect of prescribing this drug.

Now there is evidence that theophylline may be effective in lower doses than we thought. Nowadays, we have theophylline pills that are effective in a once- or twice-a-day dosage. I still see patients who take older forms of theophylline four times a day. Sometimes preparations are made in which theophylline is combined with other medications that by themselves have little effect on asthma symptoms. With these fixed-dose combinations it is usually impossible to achieve a useful level of theophylline in the blood without unacceptable adverse effects.

Professional opinion is currently divided about how useful theophylline really is in the treatment of asthma. Some think it doesn't work very well. Others think it is worthwhile in difficult situations such as in patients who get asthma attacks while sleeping. When asleep you can't use an inhaler and the effects of the beta-2 inhalers last only four or five hours. In the near future this problem may be solved by the introduction of long-acting (twelve-hour) inhaled beta-2 drugs.

**BETA-STIMULATING PILLS**   If you're still wheezing despite inhalers and theophylline, beta-stimulating pills such as Brethine or Proventil can sometimes be prescribed to further dilate your bronchi.

However, this medication does not enhance the dilation of the bronchial tubes in a person who is already inhaling a beta stimulator. And they have the possible adverse affects of making a patient feel jumpy and have a rapid heart rate.

I rarely prescribe oral beta stimulators. I would rather that the patient take more puffs of his inhalers.

**CORTICOSTEROID PILLS**   Corticosteroid pills, in the form of prednisone, are then the next step. These are the most powerful antibronchoconstrictors known.

Prednisone, however, is a double-edged sword. While it can virtually eliminate asthma symptoms in most people (as can other corticosteroids), when it is given every day in a dose higher than 10 mg there is a tendency for patients to gain weight; develop a moon face; get acne, diabetes, thin bones; and have increased susceptibility to infection. For these reasons we try to give prednisone every other day if we can. Given this way, the only adverse effect tends to be mild weight gain.

High doses of inhaled corticosteroids (which do not have these effects because they are nonsystemic) should always be tried by your doctor before starting oral prednisone. Oral prednisone takes a few hours to work. It acts to block the late-phase inflammatory response. If you are a severe asthmatic, doses of oral prednisone can keep you out of the hospital if you start to take them when you feel your inhalers failing.

## ALTERNATIVE DIAGNOSES

Sometimes all the above measures fail to help the asthmatic. It is at this point that most physicians exhaust their asthmatic armory. It is also at this point that I start rational, safe, experimental therapy. Since the effect of long-term daily corticosteroids on a patient's appearance and health are so devastating, I try to avoid them if at all possible (although every-other-day steroids, while not as effective, do not have as many adverse effects). Here are some ideas for your physician to consider.

First, has removal of environmental asthma triggers been considered? Irritant gases, cigarette smoke, domestic animals, cold air, and sulfites in foods should all be considered.

Is there an alternative diagnosis for your intermittent wheezing? Could you have been born with a malformation of the lungs or some other structure in the chest that could be reducing airflow? Could you have cystic fibrosis in a mild form? Could you be especially sensitive to a fungus called aspergillus found in dust which can cause similar symptoms? Are there symptoms of acid backing up into the esophagus from your stomach, which can produce asthmalike symptoms (see Chapter 6)? Might your lungs be filling with fluid because of congestive heart failure? Do you have a sinus infection which might be making your asthma worse?

None of these is a wonderful thing to have. But if you do, they might be causing the asthmatic symptoms—and treating them will benefit you.

Only after these and any other potential diagnoses have been ruled out do I look at innovative ways to possibly dilate the bronchi.

## ALTERNATIVE TREATMENTS

The following treatments are far from cookbook medicine but they may prove beneficial for you. If nothing else works, you may want to discuss them with your doctor.

**HYDROXYCHLOROQUINE** The drug hydroxychloroquine (Plaquenil), an anti-inflammatory drug, has been used for many years in the treatment of rheumatic disease such as arthritis and lupus. In asthma it may be useful if you've become dependent on prednisone. Prednisone taken long-term on a dally basis can have serious side effects.

I have prescribed hydroxychloroquine to asthmatics dependent on prednisone (or corticosteroid drugs) and have often found that they could at least go to alternate-day therapy. Some were able to stop corticosteroids altogether. One severe asthmatic, a forty-year-old teacher, was able to discontinue his prednisone and was actually running in marathons six months after starting hydroxychloroquine, which takes several months to have its therapeutic effect.

This use of hydroxychloroquine seems very obvious, and I reported it in a medical journal some time ago. Researchers from Australia wrote me that they had done research on hydroxychloroquine and found that it was significantly effective in laboratory studies. It is puzzling and disappointing that no asthma researchers have done a double-blind experiment to demonstrate the beneficial effects of hydroxychloroquine to the medical community at large.

Other anti-inflammatory drugs have been tried, and your doctor may wish to prescribe them for you. Some have more potential adverse reactions. Gold, sometimes used in severe arthritic conditions, has not worked. Another drug, methotrexate, has, and can be used in low doses in difficult cases. An antibiotic called triacetyloleandomycin (TAO) can reduce the required dosage of corticosteroids.

**NITROGLYCERIN**   I have prescribed nitroglycerin, used to dilate blood vessels in patients with angina, for bronchodilation in asthma and have had some success using it in children with corticosteroid-dependent asthma. Unfortunately, it does not seem to work in adults. I prescribe it in the form of patches worn on the skin so that the medicine is continuously absorbed.

A twelve-year-old boy taking daily prednisone and experiencing severe adverse effects, including weight gain, was able to stop taking the corticosteroid entirely by using a nitroglycerin patch. He is now sixteen and is growing into a tall, slim, handsome young man.

Nitroglycerin is now available (by prescription) in an oral spray that is sometimes helpful in an acute asthmatic attack. I am not aware of any other research using nitroglycerin in asthmatic children.

### DIET

Eskimos have a low incidence of asthma. They also do not have much heart disease. Both of these aspects of good health may be a result of a diet high in fish oils.

A major oil in fish is eicosapentanoic acid (EPA), one of the essential fatty acids our bodies need. Through a complex chemical process, this fatty acid can create anti-inflammatory agents in the blood. The idea is that eating more fish or taking capsules of EPA might be beneficial.

This strategy is currently being used to treat rheumatoid arthritis, high blood pressure, and, now, asthma patients. If you try it, you should probably be on a diet low in red meat, a source of saturated fatty acids, which raise cholesterol and may work against EPA.

This chemical may be purchased over the counter as Max-EPA or Pro-Mega. A derivative, docosahexaneoic acid (DHA), which may also alter production of inflammatory compounds, is included in most formulations. These treatments have not been tested very well, but seem to be fairly harmless to try. (Fish oils may be taken off the market in the near future by the Food and Drug Administration (FDA) because they have been promoted as cholesterol-lowering agents.)

# 11

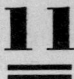

## Nose and Throat Problems

Problems associated with the nose and throat tend to go together even though they may appear to be quite different. Here we deal with both, as always trying to understand what causes the problems and the appropriate ways of dealing with them.

If you are not getting better, it may be due to the fact that your doctor is dealing with a difficult to diagnose problem and, in looking in his cookbook, isn't finding the answer. In this chapter we examine many unusual problems he may have missed. You can read this material and then compare the information with what your physician is doing and discuss with him the diagnoses and treatments suggested here.

### SORE THROAT PAIN

Just as some people think of anything wrong in the abdomen as being caused by a stomach problem, they also tend to think that any pain in the throat is caused by a strep infection. Mothers almost automatically assume, when they bring their children in with a sore throat, that it's strep—caused by a bacterium called streptococcus. If I don't automatically take a culture and prescribe penicillin, they sometimes become angry and demanding, telling me that their last doctor always gave their child a shot of penicillin when he had a sore throat.

If truth be known, only about 10 percent of all cases of sore throat are linked to a strep infection. Other causes account for the other 90 percent. There are several types of streptococcus, but only one, beta-hemolytic, is thought to cause strep throat. This doctrine has lately been challenged.

Yet many physicians still treat sore throat as strep throat, even when it's unlikely that the strep bacterium is present. I regularly see patients who complain of having multiple ''strep'' throats that are seemingly unaffected by antibiotic pills or penicillin shots.

Their lack of response is not because the streptococcus has become resistant to penicillin (it has not), but because their problem was caused by something else. As a cause of recurrent sore throat, strep throat is quite uncommon unless it was inadequately treated the first time.

In this chapter we look at some of the causes of recurrent sore throat and what can be done about them. Along the way you will get a new appreciation for what might be causing this problem. And if you're not getting better after being treated by your doctor, you'll now have some new ideas to discuss with him.

**CAUSES OF SORE THROAT PAIN**   You would think that in this age of high-tech medical marvels diagnosing so mundane a condition as a sore throat would be child's play. Yet controversies still exist about how to tell when someone has a strep throat or something else and whether it is of any value to do laboratory tests. (The tests are subject to procedural errors when the throat is scraped, as well as in interpreting the results. And they add an additional cost to the doctor–patient encounter.)

We begin by discussing strep itself, then move on to other possible causes of sore throat pain.

**Strep**   The back of the throat (the pharynx) can be the site of an infection by streptococcus bacteria. This causes a strep throat or streptococcal pharyngitis. Typically you will have an extremely painful sore throat, but lack other flulike symptoms. Symptoms may include the usual (although not invariable) appearance of redness, fever, swelling, pus, and enlarged lymph nodes in the front of the neck.

If strep throat is indeed the problem, it should clear up with a ten-day course of oral penicillin or an injection of long-acting penicillin (benzathine penicillin) or Bicillin. If the infection has worsened so that an abscess (a collection of pus) has formed, your doctor may suggest other therapy. Strep throat, however, should not be chronic. Once cleared up, it should be gone and stay away. If you are prescribed an antibiotic for ten days, take it for ten days! Most people discontinue a medication when they feel better, but the infection can recur because all the bacteria were not killed.

**Tonsillitis**     Chronic tonsillitis is a typical cause of recurrent sore throat, and your doctor should be able to come up with this diagnosis easily. Besides the sore throat, enlarged tonsils can cause problems such as sleep apnea, speech difficulties, or trouble swallowing. Chronically infected tonsils may even be a cause of bad breath.

**Treating Chronic Tonsillitis**     Although we no longer remove tonsils with the abandon of days of yore, many physicians believe that seven cases of tonsillitis in one year, five a year for two years, or three a year for three years is justification for a tonsillectomy.

Note: The administration of penicillin by your doctor may not be accurate if chronic tonsillitis is present. The fact that tonsillitis recurs even though penicillin is given suggests that it will not solve the problem, although other antibiotics might.

Other treatment options may vary among physicians. We are now learning that chronic tonsillitis may actually be caused by other bacteria (not streptococcus). As a result, I rarely refer a patient for tonsillectomy unless he or she has had a trial of amoxicillin and clavulanic acid (Augmentin) or clindamycin (Cleocin) and metronidazole (Flagyl). These antibiotics kill bacteria that would not be affected by penicillin alone. You may want to suggest this treatment to your physician.

**Viruses and Chlamydia**     I was taught in medical school that most sore throats are caused by viruses and that there is no treatment for them other than ''tincture of time.'' This maxim is generally true. However, if the sore throat is part of a flulike illness, your doctor may indeed successfully treat it with an antiviral agent, amantadine (Symmetrel). Depending on the severity of the sore throat, this may be an option you will want to discuss with your physician.

Another infectious cause, which may be relatively common, is the microorganism chlamydia. Typically it is hard to tell if these are the problem or if a strep infection is involved. Chlamydia is susceptible to antibiotics and can be treated with erythromycin or tetracycline. I prefer erythromycin because it also kills streptococcus. I often prescribe a ''shotgun'' therapy of amantadine and erythromycin for patients with sore throats that closely resemble strep.

Infectious mononucleosis can present an appearance similar to that of strep throat. You might ask your doctor if he considered this condition in his diagnosis. The symptoms of mono include severe fatigue as well as sore throat. Mono is diagnosed with a lab test and may be treated with certain medications such as Zantac or Tagamet. This treatment is not well known and has not been tested in double-blind experiments.

**NECK PAIN AS A SORE THROAT (CAROTIDYNIA)** Other causes of recurrent sore throat are not well known and are therefore frequently misdiagnosed. The most common of these is probably carotidynia, which often produces neck pain as well as a sore throat. The pain is usually one-sided and is aggravated by anything that causes the throat or the neck to move. The term *carotidynia* means that the carotid artery is painful.

Located under the midportion of the jaw, the carotid artery can be easily examined. It feels enlarged and tender in the patient with carotidynia. The diagnosis can be confirmed by pressing on the tender carotid artery from the floor of the mouth, under the tongue next to the first molar (the second tooth from the back if the wisdom teeth have been extracted). The first time I examined a patient with carotidynia I thought he had an aneurysm (ballooning-out) of his carotid artery because it was so enlarged. Laboratory tests, however, were normal. Patients usually think their enlarged carotid arteries are lymph nodes, but lymph nodes do not pulsate.

Carotidynia also seems to be related to migraine headache, because it is more common in patients who also have migraines and responds to antimigraine therapy. This problem may go away by itself after about two weeks but is sometimes chronic and recurrent. The cause is unknown, but there are no serious complications. (A disorder of arterial inflammation in the head called cranial arteritis also produces tender arteries, but the symptoms are much more severe and a lab test is usually abnormal, an elevated sedimentation rate indicating inflammation.)

**SORE THROAT CAUSED BY ACID BACKUP FROM THE STOMACH (REFLUX ESOPHAGITIS)**  Reflux esophagitis occurs when a weakening of the muscle between the esophagus and the stomach allows stomach acid to go back into the esophagus and burn it, which may cause heartburn (see Chapter 6). Sometimes the patient will complain only of a sore throat or a lump in the throat.

The physical exam is typically normal and the patient too often is treated as having a psychiatric problem, globus hystericus. Psychiatric treatment does not resolve the symptom and may make it worse if a tricyclic antidepressant, which further relaxes the weak esophageal muscle, is prescribed.

**INFLAMED THYROID**  The only symptom of an inflamed thyroid gland (thyroiditis) may be a sore throat. Unfortunately thyroiditis, though common, when it manifests as a sore throat is often missed by the physician because of failure to examine the thyroid.

Located below the Adam's apple in the front of the neck, the gland will be quite tender if there is an infection. A careful doctor can usually make the diagnosis in about five seconds, an experience that often elicits ''Why didn't my own doctor think of that?'' from a new patient. This patient will usually already have been treated with antibiotics because thyroiditis may produce a high fever and a generalized malaise.

This treatment may not be helpful because an inflamed thyroid is usually caused by a viral infection that is not affected by antibiotics. However, once the correct diagnosis is made, therapy is fairly standard. Blood tests for the thyroid antibodies and radioactive thyroid scans can be used to confirm the initial impression.

If you have thyroiditis you may have elevated or decreased levels of thyroid hormone and may have other autoimmune diseases. Thyroiditis is fairly common in Chronic Fatigue Syndrome, but is not severe.

**NERVE IRRITATION (GLOSSOPHARYNGEAL NEURALGIA)**  A stabbing, burning pain of unbearable severity on one side of the throat lasting only several seconds is the hallmark of this problem. It usually occurs in those over forty and can be recurrent for several weeks or months and then cease for a long time, only to recur.

There is usually a trigger zone in the throat that, stimulated by eating, yawning, or coughing, produces an attack. Nothing else can cause sudden throat pain that ceases abruptly and can be provoked by touching a trigger zone.

Your doctor can confirm the diagnosis by injecting the nerve with a local anesthetic and seeing if the pain is relieved. If it is, glossopharyngeal neuralgia is the problem.

Medication such as carbamazepine (Tegretol) or phenytoin (Dilantin) can usually control the symptoms.

**BONE PRESSURE**   If any disorder can be confused with nerve irritation, it is the elongated styloid process syndrome that some physicians do not think even exists.

The styloid process bone, located just beneath the earlobe, becomes a ligament that attaches to the bone in the front of the neck. When the styloid process bone is too long it can pinch the glossopharyngeal nerve or the carotid artery, producing pain.

The pain is usually constant and is made worse by swallowing. It can radiate to many areas of the mouth, head, and neck.

Your doctor can make a diagnosis by pushing on the tonsil on the affected side. This maneuver should make the pain much worse. A local anesthetic can be administered to eliminate the pain temporarily, and cortisone injected into the area can provide long-term relief, although surgery to remove the styloid process is sometimes necessary.

**INFLAMED TENDON (ACUTE CALCIFIC RETROPHA-RYNGEAL TENDINITIS)**   An inflamed tendon can cause a sore throat that is actually located behind the back of the pharynx even though this area appears normal on examination. Movement of the head aggravates this pain, and an X-ray often reveals calcification in the muscles between the back of the throat and the spine.

This condition is much like a shoulder bursitis for which patients receive cortisone injections. This area, however, is too hazardous to inject.

Your doctor can treat the pain with anti-inflammatory drugs and it usually resolves in one to two weeks. However, this syndrome may become chronic and recurrent. Fever and an elevated sedimentation rate (a blood test for inflammation) may occur.

**LESS COMMON CAUSES**  Among the less common causes of chronic or recurrent sore throat are tumors and abscesses, usually detected fairly readily by the observant physician.

Recurrent sore throat is a common symptom of Chronic Fatigue Syndrome and is sometimes encountered in patients with nasal allergy, perhaps because of post-nasal drip or because of drying of the throat due to mouth breathing and lack of humidified air.

The next time you have a chronic sore throat, don't immediately think it's strep. And don't let your doctor off the hook when he says "It's probably strep." There are a host of other possibilities.

## SINUS PROBLEMS

A stuffy nose is a problem everybody has experienced. Some unfortunate people have this difficulty only during certain seasons of the year. A few unlucky ones seem to be stopped up almost all the time.

Many of these sufferers complain to their doctors of sinus trouble or sinusitis. Yet on examination their sinuses appear normal. Countless times have I listened to a patient with a stuffy or runny nose complaining of "sinus" problems and asking me for an antibiotic.

Most of these people do not have a sinus infection but an inflammation of the nose. It could be the common cold, a form of nasal allergy, excessive nasal blockage, or discharge from other causes. The point is that in most cases the nose is the problem, not the sinus. Yet, regardless of the cause, the sinus usually gets the blame.

For your doctor, however, getting the diagnosis right can be critical to you. If it's simply a stuffy nose, an antihistamine might do. On the other hand, if it's true sinusitis, using an antibiotic treatment might be critical. Let's first consider sinus disorders, then move on to the problems of the nose.

**UNDERSTANDING OUR SINUSES**  The sinuses are hollow, membrane-lined cavities in various locations in the head.

(Interestingly enough, fish do not have them. It has been suggested that as life emerged from the oceans and had to filter air, sinuses were developed because the nose itself could not make enough mucus.)

To a minor degree, sinuses function to humidify the inhaled air and also secrete mucus. They are only noticed when they become infected or blocked. These conditions can cause various symptoms, depending on how long the disorder has been present and which sinus is involved.

Why are sinuses necessary? No one knows. The nose is much more efficient in heating, humidifying, and filtering air. There are even individuals who do not develop certain sinuses during childhood and do not seem the worse for it.

**SYMPTOMS OF SINUS TROUBLE**    Some people's sinuses become infected fairly regularly. Infection may occur when sinus openings, which drain mucus, get blocked by swelling that is often related to allergy or viral infection. Then bacteria that normally live in the sinuses in low concentrations stagnate and multiply, and patients may report a feeling of nasal congestion and pressure over the infected sinus. They may feel generally ill, have a fever (about half the time), and usually have yellow or green, often foul-smelling mucus coming out of one nostril. (The sinuses are paired, one on each side of the head; typically only one side becomes infected.)

The affected sinus may be tender, particularly if it is the maxillary sinus under the cheekbone, in which case you may feel like you have a toothache in your upper jaw. Sinusitis should be suspected if a child has frequent colds which last more than ten days.

**ETHMOID SINUSITIS**    The ethmoid sinus is located behind the eyebrow. If you have ethmoid sinusitis, the main symptom may be swelling of your eyelid on one side. You may also have localized pain as well as pain over the bridge of your nose. Ethmoid sinusitis may not hurt at first, and the swelling may be diagnosed as an allergy.

A good doctor, of course, will realize that a true allergy would usually occur on both sides, unless one eyelid had come in contact with a substance like a cosmetic or perfume that can cause the skin to become inflamed. Ethmoid sinusitis may also be misdiagnosed as an insect bite.

Misdiagnosis can result in delayed treatment, which could result in the infection spreading around the eye—a fairly serious condition. Children are especially vulnerable, since ethmoid sinusitis could spread into the brain because the bone between the ethmoid sinus and the brain is very thin in preadolescents. This condition would be critical.

**FRONTAL AND SPHENOID SINUSITIS**  The two other sinuses are above the eyebrows (frontal) and between the back of your nose and the base of the brain (sphenoid), where your pituitary gland is located. Frontal sinusitis is fairly common and can cause morning headaches that resolve after you are standing up for a while. Typically, however, they then come back later. They may hurt more when you bend over. Sphenoid sinusitis is unusual but produces a deep headache.

**WHY DO SOME PEOPLE GET SINUSITIS AND OTHERS NOT?**  The immunologic basis of why some people get sinusitis and others don't is poorly understood. The primary causes, as we understand them today, run the gamut from various kinds of mechanical obstructions to mucus drainage, including abnormal shape of the bones of the nose, bony outgrowths called spurs, tumors, and other possibly obstructing growths. In some cases the openings may just be too narrow.

**DIAGNOSING SINUSITIS**  The diagnosis of sinusitis has been made easier by CT (computerized tomography) and MRI (magnetic resonance imaging) scanners. They cost more than sinus X-rays, but a CT or MRI scan can show in much more detail what is going on. Ask your doctor about these tests if a sinus problem is diagnosed.

**Nasal Endoscopy**  Sinusitis can also be diagnosed and treated with nasal endoscopes. These are flexible telescopes, not much wider than a strand of spaghetti, that can look at the area where the openings drain as well as other surrounding structures. This procedure can be done fairly easily in a doctor's office without sedation.

Since these techniques have been available we have been

able to diagnose hitherto unsuspected sinusitis, particularly ethmoid sinusitis which in children may manifest only as a low-grade cough or nasal discharge.

**TREATMENT** Before the endoscope, many kinds of chronic sinusitis would have to be treated by operations that involved several days of hospitalization to make holes in the sinuses. Now the openings can be widened through the endoscope much as an orthopedist uses arthroscopy on a knee, and the patient can go home the same day. Endoscopic sinus surgery is probably the most significant advance in the treatment of chronic sinusitis since I became a doctor.

Before you rush out to have this procedure, however, you should know that it has been estimated that 20 percent of patients diagnosed as having chronic sinusitis actually have a problem with their upper jaws (maxillae) or with certain muscles of the jaw (lateral pterygoid). You can actually feel tenderness in these muscles by feeling behind and inside your upper back teeth. Be sure to ask your doctor about lateral pterygoid muscle pain if the sinuses behind your cheekbone (maxillary sinuses) keep hurting despite apparently adequate therapy.

If there is actually an infection of the sinus (and not a nose problem) and it is not treated in the first few days with antibiotics and decongestants, the pain may get a little better, but the nasal discharge will remain and you may become fatigued and feel generally sick. The longer the sinusitis remains, the harder it becomes to treat, since the inflammation tends to close up more and more of the draining holes that allow the mucus to flow out.

Sinuses have hairlike structures in them called cilia that move back and forth to propel the mucus toward the opening. Infection can paralyze the cilia. Smoking can also adversely affect the cilia, particularly when you have sinusitis. This is one of many good reasons not to smoke, especially when you have a cold or nasal allergy.

One of the big problems in treating with antibiotics, however, is that they sometimes aren't given long enough. They often need to be prescribed for several weeks instead of ten days as is usual for other infections. Some physicians now routinely use corticosteroid nasal sprays with antibiotics when treating chronic sinusitis. I encourage this type of therapy.

## NASAL DISORDERS

The function of the nose, besides smell, is of course to conduct inhaled air. But what most people don't realize is that the nose does other things as well, such as heating and humidifying air and filtering it so that germs and other foreign material are trapped in the mucus.

This process takes place so that the air that goes down the windpipe is at body temperature, not too dry, and relatively germ-free. Mucus from the back of the nose goes down the throat, and from the front out the nostrils. A surprising fact: Mucus itself has germ-killing properties.

**The Erectile Turbinates**   Inside the nose erectile structures called turbinates rhythmically swell or contract, depending on how much blood flow they receive. Mucus production and swelling of the turbinates are two of the main variables involved in whether you feel that your nose works properly or not. They are the reason the lower nostril gets blocked when you lie with your face to one side over a long period of time. The rhythm of expanding and contracting about every four hours is disrupted. (Try rolling over more often during the night and your stuffy nose may clear up!)

Numerous factors control the blood flow to the turbinates and mucus production, but certainly hormones are important. Pregnant women often have runny noses, and nasal problems are fairly common in menopausal women. One highly respected ear, nose, and throat specialist I know believes that too little attention is paid to hormonal supplementation and the role of alteration in the quality of the mucus in menopausal women.

**SYMPTOMS OF NASAL DISORDERS**   The relatively few symptoms of nasal disorders include:

Runny nose
Inability to smell properly
Blocked nose
Sneezing
Postnasal drip
Spontaneous bloody nose

## RHINITIS

Only a small proportion of patients who come to their doctors complaining of sinusitis actually have it. The rest have a condition called rhinitis, an inflammation of the nose, not the sinuses. Half of these have allergic rhinitis, commonly called hay fever, about which much has been learned in recent years and for which there is very effective treatment.

**ALLERGIC RHINITIS**   Patients with allergic rhinitis usually have symptoms seasonally, depending on the kind of pollen a person is allergic to. (They may also have their rhinitis all year long, if the allergy-producing material is always present.)

Patients with one allergy often have others. Asthma, eczema, and eye allergies are very common. Many of the same drugs used to treat asthma in the lungs can treat allergic rhinitis in the nose (see Chapter 10).

Itching of the eyes, nose, and back of the throat is a prominent feature of allergic rhinitis but almost never in other types. An increase in a certain white blood cell, called an eosinophil, is seen only in an allergic condition, but it is not always present. There are other tests your doctor can use, besides checking eosinophil levels, to make the correct diagnosis.

**NONALLERGIC RHINITIS**   This disorder can occur anytime (or all the time) and is not associated with itchy eyes. Postnasal drip can be overwhelming in nonallergic rhinitis. The common cold is an example of nonallergic rhinitis of short duration.

Rhinitis can also be caused by medication, using too much nasal spray, pregnancy, stress, environmental irritants, and hormone imbalances. Often we do not know the true cause (perennial rhinitis).

Rhinitis that is caused by infection but that also has increased eosinophils, which would indicate an allergic condition, is called NARES syndrome.

Sneezing is prominent in allergic rhinitis, yet when there is no increase in eosinophils in the nose but a lot of sneezing and watery nasal discharge it's called vasomotor rhinitis.

And, to make things completely confusing, there is a kind

of unclassifiable nonallergic rhinitis that is neither NARES syndrome nor vasomotor rhinitis.

**TREATMENT** Allergy shots are helpful in allergic rhinitis but have not been shown to be useful in many other disorders. There is considerable controversy about the value of allergy shots, but almost all physicians agree on their value in allergic rhinitis—all the more reason to distinguish allergic rhinitis from other types. The injections are expensive, time-consuming (once a week at the least), and painful, and take up to a year to decrease symptoms. New techniques are being developed to speed this process, and a substance called allergoid that can hyposensitize with only four to six injections a year may soon be available.

Nonallergic rhinitis can be treated with antibiotics. Corticosteroid nasal sprays (see Chapter 10) are also effective in NARES syndrome and even vasomotor rhinitis, although it is not very clear why they should be effective in the latter since there are few eosinophils present. Corticosteroids have a marked suppressive effect on these white blood cells.

**OTHER CAUSES OF RHINITIS** Other causes of rhinitis include those induced by drugs that constrict blood vessels, especially cocaine, as well as various drugs used to treat high blood pressure that block the effect of adrenalinlike substances in the body which help to decongest the nose. Birth control pills can also sometimes cause rhinitis, but this is uncommon. Nasal sprays themselves can cause the condition.

Infection can also cause rhinitis. If rhinitis is due to an infection, your doctor will see a different kind of white blood cell called a poly (polymorphonuclear leukocyte) in stained nasal secretions. He should be able to point this out to you.

If you have rhinitis in only one nostril it could be due to a tumor, polyp, or foreign body. I have spent many harrowing minutes trying to extract BBs, beans, buttons, and other such items from children's nostrils in emergency departments.

An underactive thyroid can also cause rhinitis and can be diagnosed with a common blood test.

**TREATING RHINITIS** The news here is pretty good and getting better as new types of medications become available.

However, there is no place in the treatment for antibiotics without a demonstrated infectious cause—which there usually is not.

Not too long ago all we had were antihistamines and decongestants like those you can find in Contac, Allerest, or Dristan and allergy shots.

**MEDICATIONS**   Several classes of medications are used to treat rhinitis, and others will soon be available. (Although I am going to avoid a complex explanation of the early and late phase nasal response, a technical aspect of the immune system, I will consider here the various categories of the medications used.) You may want to discuss one or more of these with your physician if you have rhinitis that is not readily clearing up.

**Antihistamines**   Nonsedating antihistamines are now available. These drugs don't get into the brain and hence don't cause you to fall asleep. One of them, terfenadine (Seldane) has been almost as widely promoted as minoxidil (Rogaine) for growing hair.

These new "third-generation" antihistamines are a significant advance. Besides Seldane, the only other one currently on the American market is astemizole (Hismanal), a very potent antihistamine that lasts a long time. (They are available by prescription only.)

You will usually be told to take Hismanal about a week before allergy season starts, or take a lot of them (three pills the first day) when you get symptoms. Hismanal needs to be taken on a regular basis, and there are reports of its effects lasting months after it was discontinued. Hismanal, as well as certain other third-generation antihistamines not yet available in the United States may also help asthma somewhat.

These medications decrease runny nose, sneezing, nasal itching, and itchy eyes but do not reverse nasal blockage very well. Hismanal may be the most effective of this type.

The new third-generation antihistamines are also remarkably free of side effects, although Hismanal has occasionally been reported to cause weight gain.

I had always been taught that if you put an antihistamine in your nose or on your skin (as in Benadryl lotion) you could become allergic to it. As a consequence I never prescribed it in itching conditions, and even discouraged my patients from using Caladryl for poison ivy. Now I'm not so sure. Some antihistamines applied in the nose appear to work quite well without side effects.

**Decongestants**  Decongestants (adrenergic antagonist drugs) have been around for a long time. Most people are familiar with pseudoephedrine (Sudafed) in its short and sustained-action form and nasal sprays such as the quick-acting Neo-Synephrine and the longer-acting oxymetazoline (Afrin) and others. These drugs offer definite benefits.

They are usually fairly well tolerated, although the pill form can make a person feel hyper and have a fast heart rate. They apparently redistribute the blood flow in the turbinates of the nose.

The nasal sprays available are only suitable for short-term use, three to five days, since they are addictive and will cause a rebound reaction when they wear off, making you more congested when they do. This type of spray should be used only long enough to decongest the nose and allow your doctor to prescribe corticosteroid sprays, which can now get past the blockage.

New adrenergic nasal sprays are being developed that may not be addictive, since they constrict the turbinates but maintain the blood flow. (Weaning people from Afrin, which, if used for an extended time, must eventually be taken every hour or so and may cause bloody noses, can be quite difficult. The corticosteroid nasal sprays are very helpful in this regard.)

**Atrovent**  Ipratropium bromide (Atrovent) is an inhaled medication used mainly in asthma, but I have been using it now and then for years in the treatment of rhinitis in which watery discharge is a prominent symptom. Take the asthma inhaler, which has a wide mouthpiece, and put the nipple of a baby bottle over it. Cut off the end of the nipple and it will fit right in your nostril. One or two puffs in each nostril four times a day should do the trick. Atrovent is usually not absorbed into the body, so side effects are minimal.

**Nasalcrom**  Sodium cromoglycate (Nasalcrom) can come in a nasal spray and is the safest nasal allergy medication avail-

able. It is also available as an eye drop for allergic itchy eyes
(Opticrom) and works fairly well for this purpose.

How Nasalcrom works is still not well understood. It is
helpful only in allergic rhinitis. It takes a week or so to work
and must be used six times a day at the beginning; later the
dose can be reduced.

**Corticosteroids**   Corticosteroids sprayed in the nose are
the best single treatment for rhinitis. They decrease the effect
of almost all related nasal problems and are not absorbed into
the body when used in the usual doses. (They are also thought
to be the best single treatment for asthma, which is increasingly being regarded as an inflammatory disorder caused in
part by eosinophil contents destroying the lining of the bronchial tubes.)

The only corticosteroid I use at present is beclomethasone
in a water base (Vancenase A/Q, Beconase A/Q); other kinds
tend to burn the nose.

The effects of these drugs may not be maximal until five to
seven days after starting treatment; a decongestant should be
used in the meantime. They are thought to be so effective,
however, that if relief of allergic rhinitis does not occur in a
few weeks and the medication is being used as directed, your
doctor should consider another diagnosis.

**Bloody Nose**   A bloody nose sometimes occurs in patients
with rhinitis. The most frequent cause is blood vessels close
to the surface in the very front of your nostrils being broken
by irritation or by wiping your nose. Home remedies such as
holding your head back and putting ice on your forehead will
not stop this bleeding. Pinching your nose for a few minutes
to compress the blood vessels usually will.

**When Medications Don't Work**   If these drugs do not
work your nasal congestion might not be due to rhinitis at all.
There are a limited number of other possibilities that your
doctor should look for:

1. There may be an anatomic abnormality in your nose such
   as a deviated septum, a tumor, or a foreign body stuck in
   a nostril.

2. An unusual kind of nasal disease called a granuloma.
3. The wrong type of drug might have been prescribed. If nasal blockage is the main symptom, decongestants and inhaled corticosteroids should be used. If a runny nose is the main problem, your doctor may try Atrovent. If the typical symptoms of allergic rhinitis are present, antihistamines should be effective.
4. There may be substances in your workplace causing the problem. No amount of treatment will help if you are continually exposed to high amounts of substances to which you are allergic.
5. It's your own fault! Noncompliance is a major reason for treatment failure. Let's face it: It is inconvenient to use inhalers up to four times a day, especially when you may need two of them. Hismanal may cause mild weight gain, and some patients will not take any medication that makes them gain weight, no matter how much it helps them otherwise. You must take the medication for it to work.
6. Smoking. If you smoke or are exposed to a lot of cigarette smoke or environmental air pollutants, you may also be fighting a losing battle. These issues must be resolved if effective treatment is to occur.
7. Incorrect use of your inhaler. Even though inhalers are very easy to use, you could still be doing it wrong, a problem that is much more common with the inhalers used in asthma. Ask your doctor to watch how you use yours to make sure you're doing it right.

With application of these principles, most patients should be greatly benefited. With our new understanding of the immunologic basis of allergic rhinitis, new treatments should be forthcoming. In many cases patients who have both allergic rhinitis and asthma note an improvement in their asthma when their allergic rhinitis is successfully treated.

# 12

## Lyme Disease

A relatively new infectious illness, Lyme disease, named after the city in Connecticut where it was first described, is causing a great public apprehension. This is particularly true in the areas of the United States where it is most prevalent—the Northeast and the upper Great Lakes region.

Part of the concern lies in the fact that the disease is so easily transmitted. It comes from a deer tick that jumps onto the skin when a person simply walks through a grassy or wooded area on a warm summer day. The environment often seems so pleasant and nonthreatening that it's hard to be wary of danger lurking there. (There were 4500 reported cases of Lyme disease in 1989, and the disease occurs on four continents. Ticks that carry the illness are spreading.)

Symptoms of the illness can easily be confused with other diseases or overlooked. This is mainly a problem in areas of the country where the tick is not yet prevalent.

In this chapter we look at what the disease is, how it is transmitted, prevention, and treatment. Along the way you will get some tips that will help you to help your doctor make a correct diagnosis.

### TRANSMISSION

Lyme disease is transmitted by a tick that feeds on human blood as part of its life cycle. This tick disgorges an infectious agent called a spirochete twenty-four to seventy-two hours after it attaches to the skin.

The tick lives primarily in grassy areas, where thousands can be present. (In these areas hundreds of ticks may attach themselves to a piece of white flannel that has been dragged across grass or underbrush for only five minutes. Can you imagine how easy it is for one of them to attach themselves to you?)

Because the tick is very small, you may not see it or recall being bitten by it.

## THE DISEASE

Lyme disease has three stages. Each stage has different symptoms.

**STAGE I** The spirochete (Borrelia burgdorferi) that causes the disease may produce a local rash (erythema migrans), the best-known symptom of Lyme disease. This rash begins as a red dot and then enlarges circularly with a central clear zone three to fourteen days after the bite.

When the rash appears, flulike symptoms may also be present. If you do not recall a rash or your doctor does not find it on a physical exam, the diagnosis of Lyme disease at this stage is very hard to make and may be missed. Most physicians do not examine a patient with the flu for a circular rash on the arms and legs unless they practice in a region where Lyme disease is common.

The first stage of Lyme disease lasts for seven to thirty-two days, after which the rash gradually disappears. There may be more than one ringlike rash in half the patients who have this disease.

The disease can be misdiagnosed in Stage 1, since the rash looks a lot like ringworm (a fungal infection) and other circular rashes. Of course, if your doctor treats you for ringworm the Lyme disease rash will not respond. Nevertheless, the diagnosis of Lyme disease may still not be made, unless, again, your doctor is in an area where the infection is common and he or she usually considers it.

An effective diagnostic technique your doctor may use is to cut off a tiny piece of the skin where the rash is located and look at it under a microscope.

**STAGE 2** The second stage occurs weeks to months later. Its main features involve the nervous system and can cause headache, stiff neck, fever, and problems in thinking: meningitis. Individual nerves may be affected anywhere in the body.

If a nerve that moves the muscles of the face is affected and deteriorates, for example, a condition called Bell's palsy may develop and one side of the face may become paralyzed. This condition usually resolves over time.

Stage 2 disease could be confused with a viral illness causing neurological symptoms, of which there are many. Heart-rhythm problems may occur in Stage 2 also, but these abnormalities are not usually dangerous.

**STAGE 3**  The third stage occurs months to years later. Its characteristics are joint inflammation and swelling (arthritis), usually of large joints like the knee; fatigue; and problems with thinking, memory, and emotions. The Lyme arthritis is the feature most people associate with the disease at this stage, although it occurs quite late in the illness.

Diagnosing the illness in Stage 3 is particularly difficult unless the patient remembers the original rash, which could have occurred months or years before. (And not everyone gets the rash.)

Even if Lyme disease is suspected, it may be hard to confirm. A blood test for the illness is available, but unfortunately the blood tests are not always reliable and results vary from lab to lab.

Even in Southern California, where I practice, some patients come to the office with a blood test indicating an exposure to the Lyme spirochete but have symptoms of Chronic Fatigue Syndrome. I must often ignore the blood test to treat their true problem.

(Many physicians now rely more on the overall clinical picture than on blood-test results. However, as noted earlier, the tendency to diagnose and treat Lyme disease is more readily made if the patient resides in an area of high Lyme disease prevalence.)

If the characteristic arthritis is present in Stage 3 the diagnosis can be made much more easily. Sometimes, however, it is not there.

## TREATMENT

The best treatment for Lyme disease is prevention, particularly if you live in an area where the illness is common.

Remember, the ticks wait in grassy areas to attach themselves to you, usually in the summertime. You should not go camping, hunting, or walking in grassy or wooded areas without having skin protection. Probably the best method is to wear long pants with the pant legs tucked into high socks. Long-sleeved shirts are also advised.

Be careful to check for ticks after you go into the woods. Keep in mind, however, that ticks may be missed after a thorough inspection, since they may be so small that it is difficult to see them with the naked eye. Light-colored clothing should be worn so that if you do get ticks you can spot them easily.

Various kinds of tick repellant are available; they should be applied to clothes, not to bare skin.

**TICK REMOVAL**   If a tick does manage to attach itself to you, you may have up to seventy-two hours to remove it before spirochetes are transmitted. Thus, you should remove it as soon as you spot it.

Contrary to popular belief, probably the best way to remove a tick is to grasp it with your fingers and pull it gently so it can be removed intact. This technique is preferable to using tweezers, heating the tick, or applying various substances, all of which may kill it but may leave a portion in your skin when you remove it.

**MEDICATION**   Lyme disease is both overdiagnosed (if a doctor relies on a blood test only) and underdiagnosed, if he or she does not think of it as a possible way to explain a clinical picture. It can also be confused with these illnesses:

Ringworm
Chronic Fatigue Syndrome
Arthritis
Viral illnesses
Lupus
Multiple sclerosis
Depression

Early treatment of Lyme disease gives the best results. Your doctor will probably use the antibiotics tetracycline or doxycycline for ten days in the early stages and for three to six weeks in the later ones. Other antibiotics may be used if tetracycline or doxycycline does not work.

If you are very ill or have not responded to oral antibiotics in Stage 2 or Stage 3, intravenous antibiotics may be used for two weeks also. This form of treatment often is effective, but sometimes not.

Unfortunately, there is no consensus on how Lyme disease should be managed by your doctor if oral and intravenous antibiotic therapy do not work.

## CATCHING LYME DISEASE FROM PETS

People concerned that they could catch Lyme disease from ticks on household pets should know that this type of transmission does not seem to occur.

## FOR THE FUTURE

You can see that the news about Lyme disease is not very good. It is difficult to diagnose if you or your doctor does not notice a rash and can be difficult to treat, especially since many of the symptoms are not caused by the spirochete directly but are a result of a response of the immune system to it.

A vaccine against Lyme disease is being developed but will not be ready for human use for several years. Until then the best approach remains prevention and early recognition.

# 13

## Mood Disorders

This chapter deals with two disorders found in every culture, country, and socioeconomic level: depression and anxiety.

It is important at the onset to discriminate between transient mood alterations and true mood disorders. At one time or another everyone is depressed or anxious. A loved one's death makes us depressed. A career in jeopardy makes us anxious. In such cases time or a change in the situation will usually resolve the anxiety or depression.

These are transient mood changes. In this chapter we go beyond them to discuss biochemically based disorders: mental states that reflect measurable changes in brain function and can incapacitate individuals.

### THE BIOCHEMICAL BRAIN

To many people and to some doctors the news that depression and anxiety disorders are rooted in biochemical imbalances in the brain is shocking. If that's the case, some might ask—if mood disorders are simply a result of a biochemical imbalance in the brain—why bother with therapy? Why not pop a pill that will correct the imbalance and be "cured?"

The answer is not simple. The brain is affected biochemically by all behavior. Experience and learning cause actual changes in the structure and function of nerve cells. Early experiences, both negative and positive, probably impoverished or enriched certain areas of our brain. These alterations produce the repertoire of our daily behaviors which in part is chemically based. The biochemical basis of behavior provides a rationale for changing mood through the use of medication. However, this is not to say that our moods cannot be modified by our attitudes, reactions, and cognitions. Our capacity to reason is very powerful, and hence the phrase *mind over matter* is an apt description of our ability to overcome many physical and emotional ailments by using our mind to change the biochemical makeup of our brain.

In short, both medication and psychotherapy affect the biochemical makeup of our brain, and both can be quite useful in treating mood disorders.

## THE PROBLEM WITH TREATMENT

If you have been diagnosed as having depression, anxiety, or another related mood disorder, a common approach is to refer you to a psychiatrist.

There are two problems with this course of action. The first is that a physical ailment could be causing you to have abnormal moods. You could be suffering from premenstrual syndrome, Chronic Fatigue Syndrome, or any of dozens of other illnesses, many covered in other chapters. Many diagnoses of mood disorders, particularly depression, are really a giant medical wastebasket. A doctor who doesn't know what's wrong may say you're depressed, particularly if you are a middle-aged woman.

The second problem is with treatment. What I propose in this chapter is a fresh approach for you and your doctor to consider. I am not disparaging psychiatry, an area in which I have some expertise. What I am criticizing are those physicians who immediately send you to a psychotherapist upon seeing a possible mood disorder.

Mood disorders can be most successfully treated with medicine in combination with psychotherapy. But for this to happen, the doctor will have to admit that the head is indeed connected to the body. In other words, a mood disorder must be considered a physical illness.

## PSYCHOTHERAPIES

Psychotherapy is quite useful in treating mood disorders, but most laypeople simply do not have any sense of the different types of psychotherapies that are available. Many people still think that a person goes to a ''shrink,'' lies on a couch, and pours out his or her innermost feelings without understanding what the psychotherapist is attempting to achieve.

Therefore let's look briefly at the philosophies behind several of the more well-accepted therapies and their general application. Then we'll examine some specific mood disorders and how they may also be treated with medication. (Remember, the combination of psychotherapy and medication is usually most effective.)

**COGNITIVE THERAPY** Cognitive therapy revolves around the idea that, by changing your thoughts about an anger- or anxiety-producing situation, you can control your stress response. The stress response is a primitive means of preserving our species in which stress triggers a "fight or flight" response. Change your thoughts about the situation and the trigger isn't pulled.

People who are depressed often have a distorted view of themselves. They may see themselves as lacking in certain attributes such as attractiveness, competence, or intelligence. Cognitive therapy holds that negative perceptions of self, the world, and the future cause depression.

On the other hand, people who are primarily anxious may view themselves as weak and unable to cope. The anxious person may remember "failure" experiences of the past, and these memories can trigger the anxiety.

The goal of cognitive therapy is to change maladaptive distortions into healthy and valid perceptions. It teaches you to view your thoughts objectively and to determine if they are based in reality.

**INSIGHT-ORIENTED THERAPY** Traditional insight-oriented psychotherapy holds that emotional problems are the basis for depression. Insight into the dynamics of the person, particularly early childhood experiences of loss and trauma, is thought to be the key to mental health.

This approach holds that just as children go through stages in their development in which they can comprehend different concepts, they also go through different emotional stages that, if disrupted, can cause conflicts later within the adult. This is the basis of psychoanalytic theory. Put simply, understand the child within you, meet that child's needs, and you will better understand why you are doing what you are doing as an adult.

To the analyst, maladaptive behaviors such as phobias (an extreme and inappropriate fear) are manifestations of internal conflict. The patient would attempt to gain insight into a current problem by examining dreams, thoughts, early experiences, and feelings. The result would be an understanding of the disrupted childhood stage and the eventual resolution of the phobia.

Unfortunately, this type of analysis is, in my view, a prolonged treatment that is prohibitively expensive. It is helpful mainly to articulate, well-to-do, educated patients willing to spend years in therapy. Some other form of psychotherapy combined with medication might produce the desired change in behavior in a much shorter period of time with much less expense.

(Various kinds of short-term ''dynamic'' or psychoanalytically oriented psychotherapies have been described as effective with depressed patients. These short-term efforts have not been subjected to as much experimental validation of efficacy, however, as have other forms of psychotherapy discussed here.)

**BEHAVIOR THERAPY**    Behavior therapy is based on principles of learning theory. In comparison to insight therapy, the time spent in treatment is minimal. Rather than analyze the psychodynamics of the behavior, the behavior itself is changed.

The reason for the learned maladaptive behavior is irrelevant in this therapy. In behavior modification the desired behavior is rewarded (reinforced) and the undesired behavior is either ignored or mildly punished. (The presence or absence of social reinforcers, environmental events the patient finds rewarding, is most often used.)

By breaking a complex behavior into small steps, the therapist shapes the desired new behavior. The patient is expected to be an active participant in his or her own therapy, defining goals and selecting reinforcers.

Behavior therapy can be used for bad habits and some addictions as well as more abstract behaviors such as fear responses (fear of driving, public speaking, and the like). Cognitive therapy is often combined with behavior therapy as cognitive-behavioral therapy.

**GROUP THERAPY**   Support systems are vital in dealing with mood disorders. We are social creatures, and the guidance and feedback of others is necessary in order to maintain an emotional balance. When a person is anxious, depressed, or ill, group therapy can provide training in appropriate socialization, offering concrete advice regarding options and validation of self.

A nonjudgmental setting in which a person can feel safe enough to share feelings with others in a similar situation can be extremely helpful in learning how to cope.

(One difference between group therapy and a support group is that group therapy has a leader trained in group dynamics while a support group, with many of the same goals, may not have a trained leader.)

**FAMILY THERAPY**   Family or couple (conjoint) therapy assumes that the family as a whole or the couple are but parts in a larger system of cultural mores and social roles that dictate behaviors. It also assumes that the depressed or anxious person usually has a ''significant other'' or a family member who also has problems.

For a person with a chronic illness or maladaptive behaviors, the impact on the family is great. Individual insight or cognitive therapy is beneficial, but changes are difficult to maintain when one goes back into an unchanged family whose members may feel threatened by changes in one of its members, even if they are positive.

Even in the most psychologically healthy of families, chronic illness (such as depression or anxiety) negatively influences family dynamics. Who better than a family member to reinforce new behaviors and offer support to a person trying to improve his life?

**INTERPERSONAL   PSYCHOTHERAPY**   Interpersonal psychotherapy is a form of psychotherapy that focuses on the relationships between the depressed patient and others, including the society as a whole. Depressed people do not relate well to others, and one component of this therapy is teaching them how to interact with others in a more effective and rewarding manner.

## WHAT IS A MOOD DISORDER?

Coming up with a simple but accurate definition is no easy chore. As an example of the difficulty, the description given in the psychiatric bible, *Diagnostic and Statistical Manual of Mental Disorders, Third Edition—Revised* (known and referred to as *DSM-III-R*) states, "The essential feature of this group of disorders is a disturbance of mood, accompanied by a full or partial Manic or Depressive Syndrome that is not due to any physical or mental disorder. Mood refers to a prolonged emotion that colors the whole psychic life; it generally involves depression or elation."

This definition is not all that helpful for me and I assume it is less so for you. It's all well and good to say that mood is an emotion that colors the psychic life, but I have trouble with the assertion that a mood disorder is a disturbance of mood that is not due to any physical or mental problem. If mood disorders are not due to a physical or mental problem, what else could they be?

Mood disorders are more common than most people suspect, and many people have them.

## MANIC BEHAVIOR

Manic behavior is not difficult to diagnose. A person who has this disorder will have a euphoric and/or irritable mood, inflated ideas about his self-worth, decreased need for sleep, and will talk very rapidly and switch topics frequently and inappropriately.

When you first meet a manic person, he may initially seem amusing if you do not know him well. He may appear to be extremely energetic and full of ideas. But soon you will come to see that his ideas are grandiose and inappropriate and that he is unable to turn them off. Everything seems to bubble out of him until you get the idea that it's not that he's excited about a particular subject or idea; it's just that he's excited.

A person who has one or more episodes of manic behavior (or the lesser form called hypomania) is technically thought to have a bipolar disorder, which for our purposes means that the mania may alternate with depression. Patients with this disorder are termed *manic-depressive.*

**HIGH ACHIEVERS**   Mania may not be all bad. Sometimes it decreases (or can be controlled) so that a milder condition is experienced. This less severe hypomania, when under control, can be seen in very productive, high-achieving individuals. A hypomanic may exert a powerful effect on other people, causing them to join him in whatever adventure he is planning. Hypomanics are often good salesmen or entrepreneurs and are sometimes described as charismatic.

**TREATMENTS FOR MANIA**   While mania is fairly obvious, hypomania may be difficult for your doctor to diagnose since it can be confused with other disorders in which it is seen. These include:

Schizoaffective behavior
Borderline personality disorder
Cyclothymia (in which mild mania alternates with mild depression)

Hypomanics tend to disregard the effect their behavior may have on others and may irritate and eventually drive away people who are self-reliant. It is very difficult to get them to enter treatment unless they also have depressed phases. (Some hypomanics have relatively few of these, but most do, especially as they get older.)

A manic mood disorder can be treated with psychotherapy, as already noted. However, treatment with medication as well is very beneficial. There was no medication effective for mania in the United States until the introduction of lithium carbonate, which revolutionized its treatment. Today other treatments for mania include carbamazepine (Tegretol), valproic acid (Depakote), and clonazepam (Klonopin).

A problem with these drugs is that if you are manic, you may not like the treatment very much. The reason is simple. When you are manic, you're "high." Taking the drug makes you feel normal. Since it is so exhilarating to feel manic and so mundane to feel normal by comparison, patients often say they feel worse rather than better.

Of course, this is not the case if your mania is so severe that it completely ruins your life. The grandiosity and impulsivity that characterize mania often result in poor life and financial decisions. If these detracting elements were not present, you might actually prefer the mood disorder. Artists, actors, and comedians are sometimes mildly manic and do not like to be treated because they feel the medication dulls their creativity and spontaneity.

If lithium is not very effective, it may be because you are what is called a rapid cycler—you quickly move from mania to depression and back again. Although lithium may help control the manic phase, it's sometimes not very effective for depression.

For the depression your doctor may want to try a type of antidepressant called heterocyclic. Other antidepressants called monoamine oxidase inhibitors (MAOIs) may be useful if the heterocyclics fail, and calcium channel blockers may help to control the mania if lithium does not. Verapamil (Calan, Isoptin) is the calcium channel blocker that has been used the most.

**Treatments for Rapid Cyclers**   If you are a rapid cycler you may actually have a kind of epilepsy in which obvious seizures do not occur. To treat your rapid-cycling your doctor may want to consider thyroid hormone in fairly low doses, particularly the kind called T3, or triiodothyronine (Cytomel). I've already mentioned the drug verapamil, but another, nimodipine, could possibly work better if yours is a difficult case, since it primarily affects the arteries in the brain.

When your doctor prescribes medication, be sure to ask him if lithium and calcium blockers are both being prescribed. They should NOT be used together; they can cause a severe adverse reaction in which you can become delirious.

Antidepressants used alone may cause a manic switch, a sudden change into mania, as may stimulants and an excessive amount of thyroid hormone, which may be prescribed in diet clinics. One of my patients rapid-cycled as part of her premenstrual syndrome and did not respond well to any treatment until I gave her danazol (Danocrine), an estrogen-blocking drug, which stopped the episodes abruptly (see Chapter 5).

**SELF-HELP**   There are also things that you can do for yourself. Probably the most important is to avoid situations that can precipitate mania. Sleep loss is one of these. (On the other hand, sleep deprivation is actually an experimental treatment for helping depression.) Be sure that you get plenty of sleep. Encourage trusted friends and family members to tell you when they perceive you are entering a manic phase. Their guidance and support may keep you from making costly mistakes while you are in a manic phase.

## DEPRESSION

A more common problem is depression without mania. Depression is so ubiquitous that it has been called the common cold of psychiatry. Almost everyone has been depressed at one time or another.

A depressive disorder, however, can be quite serious and debilitating. It can cause you to lose your job, spend your time listlessly lying in bed, and even lead to suicide.

Here I am only going to cover the types of depression that have an organic cause and are therefore treatable with drugs of one sort or another. There is also situational depression, mentioned earlier, which is caused by life experiences such as grief and loss. Situational depression can be treated with psychotherapy alone, but if it persists for an extended time, antidepressants may be effective. As we understand more about the biology of depression, we may discover that the distinctions between situational and organic depression are artificial.

**SEVERE DEPRESSION**   With this problem (called major depressive disorder), a person is depressed almost all of the time. In children or adolescents the depression may manifest itself as irritability. Depressed adults are apathetic, have a significant weight loss or gain, and sleep excessively or have insomnia. They may be agitated or slowed down in their movements and feel fatigued almost all the time, although this fatigue does not translate into decreased exercise tolerance. In other words, they may not want to exercise but are able to do so when encouraged or forced to and often feel a little better afterward.

If you have a major depressive disorder you feel inappropriately worthless and guilty. It will be difficult for you to think or concentrate, although if you are neuropsychologically tested and encouraged during the testing, you will do reasonably well. Your cognitive skills remain basically intact. You will tend to think about death a lot, often about suicide. You may try to kill yourself.

If you have a friend or relative who is deeply depressed, it's important to help him out; he may not be able to help himself. Severe depression is a serious illness; you should try to get him to a physician who can determine if he needs to be hospitalized. Don't let a doctor dismiss depression out of hand. If he recommends that your friend or relative see a psychiatrist, do it quickly. Left untreated, severe depression can and sometimes does lead to the tragic consequence of suicide.

**TREATING SEVERE DEPRESSION**  People with severe depression may need to be hospitalized. Hospitalization can protect them from suicidal impulses. Drugs and psychotherapy can alleviate the depression. A milder form of depression called dysthymia does not usually require hospitalization.

A medication typically prescribed is fluoxetine (Prozac), probably the most widely used antidepressant at the time of this writing. Although there has been much publicity about adverse reactions to this drug, including increases in depression and aggressive behavior, the instances are rare and the drug is still a useful one.

## DELUSIONS AND HALLUCINATIONS

Mood disorders can have bizarre symptoms. Hallucinations or delusions are symptoms of a very severe depression or a schizoaffective disorder. (Of course, if you are having a delusion, you won't recognize it. Parents, family, friends, and a good doctor may be able to help you if you let them.)

People with this disorder often don't tell their doctors. If you have a problem that you believe is real, mention it. More important, if your doctor doesn't ask, bring it up. If you have a relative or friend who has such a problem, bring it to the doctor's attention. Don't assume that your doctor knows. He can't read minds.

## DEPRESSION IN A BORDERLINE
## PERSONALITY DISORDER

Sometimes the depression you see in a friend or relative is more than just an abnormal mood; it may actually be an aspect of borderline personality disorder.

With this problem the depressed person is also very demanding, manipulative, and hard to get along with no matter what you try. He may be quite impulsive, easily angered, and may have attempted suicide or threatened to do so on seemingly little provocation. He cannot maintain stable relationships and is continually disappointed because he expects so much of others.

**TREATMENT**   You may find it difficult to find a doctor who will treat this person. Most physicians find them extremely stressful.

I have had several patients like this. One who had chosen to have me as her doctor for many years because she also has some unusual medical disorders was extremely demanding of my attention, and I would get 2:00 A.M. suicide calls at least two or three times a year.

Psychiatrists I referred her to always found some reason to refer her back, and she never liked them as much as she liked me, at least when she was not hating me because she felt I had somehow let her down. After her third or fourth potentially lethal suicide attempt she had used up the lifetime psychiatric benefits of her insurance and could no longer afford psychiatric attention. I was getting desperate for a solution to her problem.

Through the use of a BEAM scan I found that she showed some temporal lobe (brain) abnormality possibly related to epilepsy. Her BEAM scan was so abnormal I thought she should have experienced a seizure, but she had not. Sometimes patients with borderline personality disorders have temporal lobes that do not function properly.

Treatment was now possible. I quickly put her on a drug called Tegretol, which is used in certain types of temporal lobe problems. This intervention was about a year ago, and she now deals with her problems more appropriately. I haven't lost a night's sleep over her, either on the phone or in the intensive care unit, since that time.

In her case, treatment was possible because testing revealed physical abnormalities in the brain. However, when the tests are normal, there may be no good pharmacologic treatment for borderline personality disorder. Even if you have not had a BEAM scan or a similar study, your doctor may still try carbamazepine (Tegretol) or valproic acid (Depakote), medicines that affect the temporal lobes of the brain.

If you are a friend or relative of someone with borderline personality disorder, you may have to keep moving from doctor to doctor until you find one who is willing to put up with all the stress he or she can cause.

## MOOD DISORDERS AND
## CHRONIC FATIGUE SYNDROME

The last issue we will deal with while discussing mood disorders is Chronic Fatigue Syndrome (CFS), which was discussed in detail in Chapter 4. However, since many CFS patients also exhibit mood disorders, it's also appropriate to mention that aspect of the disease here.

If you have CFS, you may be chronically fatigued and have memory problems and sleep disorders. When you go to the doctor, you may be misdiagnosed as having a mood disorder, probably either major depressive disorder or dysthymia.

CFS patients are depressed because of the effect of the disease on their brains or because they are chronically ill and cannot function well. They feel rejected by doctors and sometimes by friends and family who do not understand what is wrong with them. The fact that their symptoms sometimes respond to antidepressants makes things even more confusing to those who are trying to understand how the disease works.

**CFS AND DEPRESSION**   It is important that your doctor be able to distinguish between depression as a primary disorder and depression as a symptom of CFS. The distinction is fairly easy to make; you can probably make it yourself.

If you have CFS you will exhibit most of the following symptoms, which will not be present in regular depression: fatigue made worse by exercise, chronic sore throat, marked intolerance of alcohol, nasal allergies, muscle pain, vertigo, marked thinking difficulties (poor memory, for example). Often these symptoms have a sudden onset.

In addition, when you are examined, your doctor may be able to detect other characteristic symptoms of CFS not associated with depression. These include: tender points in muscles found in the disorder called fibromyalgia (see Chapter 1), poor balance, and occasionally an unusual obliteration of fingerprints. There are also abnormalities in immune cell function and neuropsychological test results. Functional brain imaging techniques that create visual images of how the brain is working (BEAM, PET, and SPECT scans) can distinguish depressives from those with CFS. The most reliable biologic test for depression, the corticotropin releasing hormone (CRH) test, is normal in CFS patients even though they may feel depressed.

If you have classic depression you will have a more rapid onset of REM sleep than normal and have more of it. CFS patients have delayed REM sleep and have a different sleep disorder affecting NREM sleep (called alpha-delta).

Treating depression due to CFS is different from treating classic depression. Antidepressants are used, but usually in smaller doses. A most dramatic treatment—when effective—is intravenous gamma globulin, which can lift CFS depression in an hour while relieving other symptoms as well.

I've gone to great lengths to stress the measurable differences between classic depression and a depressed CFS patient mainly because so many doctors today refuse to recognize CFS. Instead they simply fasten onto the symptom of depression and leave it at that. As I have said, depression has become the great medical wastebasket. When the doctor doesn't know what's wrong with you, too often he will write down *depression* and pass you off to the next doctor, who may do the same thing. You, of course, don't get better.

If you suspect that in addition to feeling depressed, you also have other symptoms not associated with depression, reread Chapter 4 and talk to your doctor about it. If he pooh-poohs the disorder, your only recourse is to find a more enlightened doctor.

Psychotherapy, particularly group therapy led by a psychologist, is a great aid for those with CFS-related depression. If no group therapy is available, a CFS support group will be helpful.

## SEASONAL DEPRESSION

Many people are depressed in the late fall and winter months only. (Some people get depressed only in the summertime.) These patients have seasonal affective disorders and the acronym is appropriate: SAD.

Seasonal depression does not by itself indicate a primary mood disorder. It is seen as a part of other illnesses, notably sleep disorders and CFS. Seasonal depression is probably caused by a malfunction of your circadian pacemaker. This pacemaker is the part of the body that follows a twenty-four-hour rhythm and controls sleep, among other things. A circadian malfunction can also affect the part of the brain that regulates emotions, the limbic system. If you have seasonal depression, you will typically oversleep and crave carbohydrates. You may also gain weight and withdraw socially.

**TREATING SEASONAL DEPRESSION**   Seasonal depression responds well to bright light therapy for one to five hours a day. Using a special sun lamp is one of the ways you can get bright light when the sun isn't shining.

Simply basking under a sun lamp with protective eyeshades won't do, however. The exposure must involve the eyes and not just the skin. However, the eyes must be protected from too much light or they will be damaged.

This type of depression also is responsive to such drugs as tranylcypromine (Parnate) or Prozac. These agents can reduce or eliminate the necessity of light therapy.

## ANXIETY

It's hard to live in today's world and not feel anxious. If it's not conflict in the Middle East, it's gang warfare in the central city. At home we may have troubles with our children, marital problems, financial difficulties, and a host of other stresses. Is it any wonder most of us feel anxious?

And yet, there is a difference between those of us who occasionally feel anxious about things and then cope and those of us who have anxiety attacks or are generally anxious and disabled by a pervasive dread. It's sometimes a fine line to draw, but when our anxieties themselves start influencing the rest of our lives, we should realize that something's wrong. Maybe the anxiety is not just related to life events but could be produced inappropriately.

**WHAT IS ANXIETY?**  Biologically, anxiety disorders may be related to dysfunction of the limbic system of the brain. An emerging hypothesis is that this limbic dysfunction may be genetically pre-determined and affected adversely or beneficially by experience. A primary function of the limbic system is to regulate emotional responses.

You may have already experienced one or more of the various kinds of anxiety disorders that we are prone to. These might include an anxiety or panic attack, obsessive or compulsive behavior, or simply a general feeling of unrest.

You may even realize that anxiety is related to a primal feeling of fear. In nature anxiety would help to mobilize man against a threat either from an attacker or from separation from his group. In this sense anxiety, at one point in human development, was adaptive or essential to survival.

The problem, however, is that today our complex lives give us all sorts of input that arouse fears of an attack (such as a challenge to our job by a fellow worker) or fear of separation (as when we have an argument with a spouse or an employer). The anxiety that was once so essential to our moment-to-moment survival in a hostile environment can now get in the way of dealing with our daily modern stress.

**SYMPTOMS OF ANXIETY**  If you have had excessive feelings of upset, uncertainty, worry, or fear of a real or imagined danger for more than six months about two or more of life's situations such as job or marital stability, health, the economy, or people's opinion of you, plus at least six of the following symptoms, you could have a generalized anxiety disorder. (This list is adapted from *DSM-III-R*, the diagnostic manual of psychiatric disorders.)

*Motor tension sensations* such as shakiness or trembling, muscle aches, difficulty keeping still, becoming tired easily.
*Nervous system overactivity* such as sweating, dizziness,

nausea or diarrhea, hot or cold flashes, shortness of breath or shallow breathing, irregular or rapid heart rate, dry mouth or trouble swallowing.

*Hypervigilance* manifested by a feeling of being "wired" or keyed up, becoming startled easily, irritability, insomnia or difficulty falling asleep, problems in concentrating.

Remember, we all experience one or more of these symptoms at one time or another. However, if they become chronic or so intense that they affect our lives in a dramatic way, they are a disorder that needs treatment.

## DOCTOR FAILURE TO TAKE ANXIETY SERIOUSLY

Many physicians dismiss anxiety as a treatable disorder because they think that it really doesn't happen very often. While they are willing to accept depression as a common problem, and indeed seem willing to blame it for virtually every illness they cannot otherwise diagnose, they are frequently unwilling to diagnose anxiety. (Depression and anxiety, of course, often coexist in the same person.)

Further, even when they are willing to deal with anxiety, many doctors misdiagnose the disorder because it has so many manifestations, some of which we discuss in the remainder of this chapter.

Use this chapter as a guide. If you feel anxious and go to your physician and he doesn't help reduce your anxiety or, worse, dismisses your feelings saying that they don't exist when you know very well that they do, you should compare what I've written with what your physician has said. Explain to him that your problems are real and you deserve treatment.

## CONDITIONS THAT CAN PRODUCE ANXIETY    First,

let's look at a list of some of the illnesses that can produce anxiety as a symptom. Ask your doctor whether he or she has eliminated them as a cause of your anxiety. If you have one of these problems, you may find that as soon as the illness is treated the anxiety goes away.

Chronic Fatigue Syndrome (CFS)
Hormone problems, including hyperthyroidism and
   hypoglycemia
Overactivity or tumors of the adrenal gland
Inner-ear problems causing vertigo
Neurologic disorders
Partial complex epileptic seizures
Premenstrual syndrome (PMS)
Rapid heart rate
Rare tumors
Withdrawal from sedatives or antianxiety medications

**DRUGS THAT CAUSE ANXIETY**   A number of drugs can
also produce anxiety. Did you start feeling anxious just recently? Did you begin taking any of the following drugs at
about that time? If so, ask your physician if there is a
connection.

*Cocaine*
*Caffeine.* Many people who drink six to eight cups of coffee
   a day do not realize they are drinking so many and can't
   imagine why they feel anxious. Reducing or eliminating
   the coffee intake may almost immediately eliminate the
   anxiety.
*Decongestants* such as pseudoephedrine (Sudafed).
*Theophylline*, used to treat asthma. (A good antidote for too
   much theophylline is one of the benzodiazepines, one of
   the primary drugs used to treat anxiety.)
*Thyroid medication* in excess

## PANIC ATTACKS

A panic attack is a special kind of anxiety. Panic attacks are
fairly common. When they are recurrent or when a patient
worries that they may recur, a panic disorder is said to exist.
A panic attack usually comes unexpectedly and lasts a few
minutes to an hour or two.

What is peculiar about a panic attack is that the symptoms
you experience can be severe, yet they are not related to

anything you are worrying about at the time. The panic episode usually, but not always, begins with a sudden feeling of terror or impending doom. You may experience choking sensations, shake, or tremble. You may fear going crazy or even fear dying. Frequently, in my practice the degree of anxiety experienced is considerably less than the severity of the symptoms.

Episodes of anger that have no apparent cause may actually be a variation of a panic attack. They have been called, appropriately, anger attacks.

**RELATED PHYSICAL PROBLEMS**   In addition to the psychological discomfort, panic attacks may also produce related physical problems:

> *Chest Pain.* Panic disorder may cause chest pain by constricting the small arteries in the heart and causing decreased blood flow. You should never assume, however, that chest pain is only caused by anxiety; it could be a heart attack (see Chapter 8).
>
> *Hyperventilation.* Breathing too deeply and too fast may cause some of the symptoms seen in a panic attack, such as shortness of breath, numbness, tingling, and faintness.
>
> *Vertigo.* Many people state that they feel anxious because they have vertigo. However, usually the vertigo is a symptom of the anxiety.
>
> *Nausea, Vomiting, Diarrhea, and Abdominal Pain.* These are also frequent symptoms of generalized anxiety as well as of a panic attack. Patients with irritable bowel syndrome often have anxiety disorders.

**ANTICIPATING YOUR ANXIETY**   After you have a few panic episodes you may begin to worry about when the next one will occur. This phenomenon is actually a recognized disorder of its own called anticipatory anxiety. It has been speculated that this condition can lead to agoraphobia (literally, fear of open spaces), which may arise from not wanting to be in a situation from which one could not escape in case a panic attack should occur.

**TREATING YOUR PANIC DISORDER** The best treatment for panic disorder is behavioral therapy, specifically cognitive-behavioral therapy, since it's much easier for you to change your beliefs and behavior than it is to change your mood. That means that the therapy focuses not on recollecting your childhood traumas but on dealing directly with your problem. Most people who receive cognitive-behavioral therapy report they are able to control their anxiety.

Unfortunately, many insurance plans do not cover therapy and many people simply cannot afford to pay for it. An alternative is therefore to find a support group that is specifically for those with anxiety disorders. Call your local public health department for a referral.

In conjunction with behavioral therapy or the help of a support group, your doctor may suggest certain drugs that alleviate anxiety.

**Drug Treatments for Panic Disorder** You may want to discuss these medications with your doctor; they can only be taken under his supervision. Drugs that might be prescribed for panic disorder include: antidepressants such as nortriptylene (Pamelor) and fluoxetine (Prozac) as well as clonazepam (Klonopin). Klonopin is used because it has a long duration of action, is an anticonvulsant, and the withdrawal symptoms when it is discontinued are less severe than other drugs of its class (benzodiazepines). A legitimate concern about addiction to these kinds of drugs has increased the popularity of another drug, buspirone (Buspar), as an antianxiety medication that is not habit-forming. Unfortunately, it is not very effective in treating panic disorders.

Some other drug alternatives in the treatment of anxiety disorders may not have been considered by your doctor. If the symptoms of the anxiety disorder are mainly physical, propanolol (Inderal) may be helpful. Inderal is also useful in performance anxiety and is sometimes taken by those who suffer acute anxiety before public speaking, musical performance (especially by violinists, for whom hand tremor could impair performance), and before important examinations.

Calcium channel blockers sometimes have antianxiety effects and may work when other drugs have not. I first described this effect several years ago, and my work has been confirmed by others.

I have used an anticonvulsant named valproic acid (Depakote) to treat anxiety disorders that did not respond well to anything else. It seems to work in both generalized anxiety disorder and panic disorder. In anxiety disorder related to epilepsy—some seizures have anxiety as a manifestation—carbamazepine (Tegretol) and phenytoin (Dilantin) are effective.

There can be several causes of vertigo, a sensation that one's surroundings are moving or spinning. Most of these involve the organ of balance in the inner ear. Often no cause is found and a motion-sickness remedy like Antivert can prove helpful. Other ways of reducing vertigo involve niacin (to increase inner-ear blood flow) and allergy treatment. Vertigo as a symptom of an anxiety disorder usually resolves itself when the anxiety is successfully treated.

Another drug with possible anti-anxiety effects is octreotide (Sandostatin). I discovered this when I was using it to treat patients with fibromyalgia, a disorder causing muscle pain; many of them also had generalized anxiety disorder and some had panic disorder. Some reported that their anxiety was greatly reduced, or gone, while the drug was given.

## OBSESSIVE COMPULSIVE BEHAVIOR

*Obsessions* are recurrent intrusive thoughts, impulses, or images. Most kinds of nondrug therapy don't work for obsessive compulsive disorder, but certain kinds of behavior therapy are helpful, especially in conjunction with medication.

*Compulsions* are repetitive acts performed to ward off some dreaded consequence that you do not really know but are sure you don't want to happen. The person who performs compulsive actions realizes that they are excessive and unreasonable but becomes very anxious if he resists them. The anxiety is immediately relieved when the compulsion is yielded to, only the need to perform it builds up again.

The really unfortunate problem with obsessive compulsive behavior is that when someone who has the problem finally drums up enough courage to admit it to a physician, the doctor may not realize it should be taken seriously and may simply dismiss it. In this case you would be far better off with a referral to a psychiatrist trained in behavioral therapy.

Obsessive compulsive disorder was once thought to be rare. Recent surveys have indicated, however, that at least a million Americans have this problem, possibly more. I have included it with anxiety disorders since it causes distress and, if a person has compulsions, he becomes extremely anxious if he cannot perform them.

**ARE YOU OBSESSIVE COMPULSIVE?** It's important to understand the difference between becoming occasionally obsessed and feeling compelled to do something. If you have a song you can't stop thinking of, or a compulsion to arrange things in a certain order and you quickly get past it, it's probably not something to be concerned about. On the other hand, when obsession or compulsion persist and significantly interfere with your life, they should be treated.

One of my patients took seven or eight showers a day because he kept feeling that he was getting dirty in various ways. It took courage on his part to admit the problem, which had been bothering him. Once he admitted it, however, it was possible to begin treatment.

Another common compulsion is "checking." Most of us have had the experience of leaving the house and wanting to go back to make sure we turned off the stove or a similar worry. Checkers keep going back again and again. I treated one woman who worried whenever she went over a bump in the road that she had hit a pedestrian or a dog. She would go back to look and, not seeing anything, drive away, only to wonder whether she looked hard enough and drive back again.

**WHAT CAUSES OBSESSIVE COMPULSIVE DISORDERS?** Compulsive behavior is thought to be genetic, since it involves parts of the brain that are related to certain survival behaviors: grooming, in the case of cleanliness compulsions, or the need for vigilance in the case of checking.

Obsessions are also genetically based. They may be violent or unpleasant thoughts that are usually neutralized and kept from our consciousness by a part of the brain, the corpus striatum. If for some genetic reason this part of the brain is not developed properly, these thoughts are not suppressed automatically and you must consciously try to control them, an effort that results in continuing anxiety and tension.

It is striking that obsessive compulsive behaviors are remarkably similar from culture to culture and are one of the few psychiatric disorders in which the symptoms are the same in both children and adults.

**THE WRONG DIAGNOSIS**   Your doctor's failure to correctly diagnose obsessive compulsive disorder (OCD) is often not oversight on his part but simply a matter of not looking for the problem. Asking questions about these kinds of symptoms is usually not part of your doctor's initial diagnostic evaluation. On the other hand, it probably should be if you exhibit anxiety, depression, or Tourette's syndrome (see Chapter 14), since these problems are often accompanied by obsessive compulsive behavior.

If you are concerned about an obsessive compulsive behavior, put aside your embarrassment and divulge this secret so that you can be treated.

**TREATING OBSESSIVE COMPULSIVE DISORDER**
I have seen many patients with obsessive compulsive disorder over the years, and until recently treating them has been quite frustrating for me. When the drug fluoxetine (Prozac) was introduced, this disorder became more amenable to treatment, yet Prozac worked in some patients but not in others. For those in whom Prozac was unacceptable, I've tried, with limited success, trazedone (Desyrel) and MAOIs.

Now a drug that has been used to treat obsessive compulsive disorders in virtually every country in the world is finally available in the United States. This drug, clomipramine (Anafranil), helps many of those not helped by Prozac.

# 14

## Problems Originating in Childhood

This chapter is about behavioral problems—disorders not covered in the rest of this book and not well understood by some doctors, including:

Tics
Conduct disorder
Depression in childhood
Anxiety disorders of childhood and adolescence
Hyperactivity
Bedwetting

These problems usually originate in childhood and are thus most often associated with children, although they may be seen in any age group. They can be extremely difficult for parents to handle as well as difficult or embarrassing for the person who has them. Further, their diagnosis can be difficult for those doctors who only use the cookbook.

My goal, here as elsewhere in this book, is to give the lay reader a clearer understanding of what may be causing certain behavior disorders and what should be appropriate treatment. Then you can compare this information with what your doctor has said and done. This process should give you a concrete basis for deciding whether or not your doctor might be wrong. You can then ask him or her about your concerns.

## TICS

Many people experience tics at one time or another. Often under stress people find themselves blinking involuntarily or making a little sound in the throat. These repetitive behaviors may disappear as soon as the stress leaves. Sometimes, however, tics can be a long-lasting and serious problem. Your doctor may have little knowledge of tic disorders and not know how to manage them.

Tics are basically irresistible behaviors (although they can be suppressed for a period of time): A patient feels he simply must perform them. They vary greatly from a simple vocal tic, when someone feels compelled to make a noise or a grunt, to complex tics, when an affected person utters words or even sentences.

There are also simple motor tics, such as blinking or shrugging, and complex motor tics that involve many different movements. Usually they involve either a motor disorder or a grunt or vocal disorder, but not both. All tics are generally rapid and repetitive.

Tics may be short-lived, lasting less than twelve months, or chronic, lasting more than twelve months and sometimes for a lifetime. A chronic motor or vocal tic lasting more than twelve months is called Tourette's disorder or Tourette's syndrome and is named after the French physician who described the condition more than a hundred years ago.

Tics develop from stress or sometimes as the result of medications used to treat attention deficit/hyperactivity disorders. Sometimes the cause remains a mystery.

**TREATING TIC DISORDERS**   Tic disorders can be difficult for your doctor to treat. Sometimes they are associated with attention deficit/hyperactivity disorders (discussed later in this chapter) and the medications used to treat one can adversely affect the other.

The most common treatment involves the use of a group of drugs called neuroleptics. Those most commonly used are haloperidal (Haldol), pimozide (Orap), fluphenazine (Prolixin).

You should be aware of some possible severe adverse reactions to these medications. Sometimes physicians overlook them. You should promptly bring them to your doctor's attention if they occur.

One adverse reaction is smacking movements of the lips and tongue and jerking or twisting movements of the arms and other parts of the body called tardive dyskinesia. Sometimes when the drug is discontinued, the problem goes away. But sometimes it does not, and treatments for this are not very effective. About ten years ago I saw several board-certified psychiatrists who did not recognize tardive dyskinesia in a hospitalized patient, instead calling it hysterical behavior. Fortunately, this error would be much less common today.

Another adverse reaction to neuroleptics occurs when the affected person develops a fever, his heart rate goes up, he perspires, his muscle enzymes increase (implying damage to the muscles), he becomes mute and delirious or has kidney damage; in some cases he may die. The problem is called neuroleptic malignant syndrome and is serious.

If your doctor fails to recognize the problem for what it is but thinks it's a worsening of a misdiagnosed psychosis, he may prescribe even more neuroleptics. This only jeopardizes the patient affected even more.

On the other hand, besides the doctor who may not recognize an adverse reaction caused by neuroleptics, there is the doctor who is aware of the potential problems and therefore refuses to prescribe them at all. Typically this physician will give these drugs only for the most severe cases of Tourette's syndrome.

Caution with neuroleptics is necessary. In mild to moderate cases I have found another group of drugs called calcium channel blockers to be quite effective. These include verapamil (Calan, Isoptin) and nifedipine (Procardia).

I was the first to describe this treatment, using Procardia, the only calcium channel blocker available at the time. A mother brought in her thirteen-year-old son Barry because his psychiatrist said he had hysteria and she thought he had nothing to be hysterical about.

She was right: He was jerking his head and grunting quite frequently. She did not want him to take Haldol for reasons just mentioned, or another drug, clonidine, because it can cause depression and low blood pressure.

However, calcium channel blockers are relatively free of

adverse reactions and for various neurochemical reasons I thought they might work. With the consent of his mother, Barry took the Procardia. Thirty minutes later his Tourette's disorder stopped.

It never recurred as long as he took the Procardia. "We always know when it's time for Barry to take his pill," his mother commented on one of their follow-up visits. The efficacy of this treatment has been confirmed by other investigators and should be brought to the attention of your doctor if he is unaware of it.

Procardia, however, does not always work alone. Sometimes a combination of a calcium channel blocker and a neuroleptic will be effective together when neither is effective singly.

## CHILDREN WHO BREAK SOCIETY'S RULES

Bad behavior is common, at various times, among all children. However, occasionally the bad behavior is extreme, something other than "just a phase he's going through."

I'm speaking of chronic behavior that involves stealing, lying, fighting, being cruel, and getting in trouble with the law. Substance abuse is commonly seen, and there are often relatives with histories of antisocial behavior and jail sentences. Called conduct disorder, this behavior is defined technically as "a persistent pattern of conduct in which the basic rights of others and major age-appropriate societal norms or rules are violated" by *DSM-III-R*.

Children behave this way for many reasons, from genetic predisposition to lack of adequate parenting to the joining of gangs, where the behavior may be viewed as conforming to group norms.

Conduct disorder sometimes occurs by itself, but often it is seen in association with depression and hyperactivity.

**TREATING CONDUCT DISORDER**   If you have a child with conduct disorder, I don't need to tell you that he or she is extremely difficult to deal with, let alone to treat. Medically speaking, getting these children to follow a course of treatment can be nearly impossible, since not following rules or caring about what their parents or doctor says is par for the course.

I can easily recall the days when virtually all of these children were said to be acting out: expressing unconscious conflicts related to mistreatment by their parents or neglect of some sort. Although this opinion may have been true in certain children, this notion has made too many parents feel guilty and has not enabled them to be detached enough to set firm limits in the manner necessary to control the behavior.

While the tendency among parents is to believe that the disorder is caused by something they did (or did not do) while raising the child, I believe it is largely genetically based, specifically with regard to abnormalities in the activity of the frontal lobes of the brain, which regulate impulse control. Dysfunctional families can, however, cause and perpetuate many childhood behavior disorders.

Beware of being referred to therapists who want to use insight-oriented psychotherapy as a treatment. This form of treatment is not appropriate for the child with conduct disorder, since it may help him rationalize his behavior, blame others for it, and perhaps not change it.

Ideally treatment would be multimodal. A patient should have a comprehensive diagnostic evaluation, family therapy, behavioral therapy, medication, and possibly, in severe cases, even hospitalization for a period of time. (There should also be more brain-imaging done in these children. Frontal- and prefrontal-lobe dysfunction is commonly seen on BEAM and SPECT scans and can aid in diagnosis as well as suggesting treatment.)

The best medical treatment for impulse-control disorders of all sorts, including conduct disorder, remains lithium carbonate, a drug that is greatly underutilized in children. If certain precautions are taken, it is quite safe and can be used for many years. Unfortunately, there seems to be a general reluctance on the part of child psychiatrists to use medications to alter behavior, and many parents have brought their children to me in desperation after three to six months in a psychiatric hospital with no medication even prescribed and the child just as impaired as when he or she went in. Not all, maybe not even most, children with conduct disorder will be helped by lithium, but some will benefit greatly.

**DEFIANT CHILDREN** Children with conduct disorder tend to try to violate societal norms without getting caught. In many ways, they are like criminals on the loose. On the other hand, others prefer to defy authority blatantly no matter what the consequences are. They have short tempers and consistently confront authority figures. They refuse to obey adults or to do chores or perform similar obligations. They aren't concerned with getting caught. (This problem is called oppositional defiant disorder.)

Some physicians think both disorders are simply variations of the same problem. Oppositional defiant disorder is thought by some to be a less severe form of conduct disorder. Perhaps it is, in certain children. In my experience, however, they seem to be different problems.

Often the difference is fairly easy to spot; the classic conduct-disorder child will try to con you and seem to have no conscience whatsoever. The defiant child is oppositional and obnoxious. Children with both types of disorder do not seem to learn by experience and continue to engage in the same behaviors no matter how often they are caught and punished. Reward systems, if they work at all, are effective only as long as they are in effect.

My most vivid memory of the child who is disruptive in his behavior will always be angelic-looking six-year-old Eddie. Eddie did not want to leave the waiting room to come into my office, so I went out to see him, his mother long ago having abandoned any disciplinary efforts. In a firm but kind voice I told (not asked) Eddie to come into my office.

"———you!" Eddie yelled, and I knew that the rest of my diagnostic evaluation would just be window-dressing. Fortunately, children with oppositional defiant disorder frequently respond to antidepressants, and four weeks later Eddie had turned from Dr. Jekyll, Jr., into a rather normal little boy, which he remained as long as he took his medicine.

Untreated, some children with conduct disorder become what we used to call juvenile delinquents but are now described as having an antisocial personality. This topic is complicated, but one aspect of it is that these children seem to have no conscience. Their behavior often persists into adulthood.

**TREATING DEFIANT CHILDREN**   Behavioral therapy may simply not work here, at least not by itself. Check with your doctor to see if he or she is willing to prescribe an antidepressant. Children with defiant disorder sometimes respond to antidepressant treatment alone. (Interestingly enough, children with conduct disorder usually do not.)

## DEPRESSION IN CHILDHOOD

It was once believed, by laypeople and psychoanalysts alike, that children could not become depressed. The psychoanalysts felt that children did not have sufficient superego development to allow depression.

I always had trouble with this notion, because it was obvious to me—and anyone else who looked—that children do indeed become depressed. Therefore, in spite of this commonly held belief, I gave antidepressants to sad, withdrawn children—and they got better. Even today, this practice may still be controversial, although quite a bit less so, since children have been shown to have some of the biochemical abnormalities that depressed adults have. Yet a few doctors persist in dismissing depression in children. Many still feel it is not very common.

**DETERMINING WHEN A CHILD IS DEPRESSED**  It is difficult for a child younger than seven or eight to tell you that he is sad. Children of this age and younger do not have the cognitive development that enables them to express their feelings this way. They really need to be quite a bit older, perhaps midadolescent, before they are able to, in a sense, stand outside themselves and observe their behavior and what its consequences are. When they are very young, they act as their thoughts or feelings dictate.

Childhood and adolescent illnesses that may be confused with depression include:

Over- or underactive thyroid
Anemia and iron deficiency
Other hormonal problems
Premenstrual syndrome
Chronic Fatigue Syndrome
Cancer
Hyperactivity
Neurologic disorders

Viral illnesses
Drug withdrawal
Anxiety disorders

Depressed children, even when they are very young, give off many clues you can look for. They may engage in self-mutilating behavior, pulling out their hair or biting their skin. They might be accident-prone. They may have a variety of other problems—problems in school, temper tantrums, cruelty to pets. They often have impaired peer-group relationships. You should be suspicious if there is a family history of depression. Also, be aware that depression could be a symptom of some other psychiatric disorder. When in doubt, your doctor can run some psychological tests that can detect depression in a child.

Some authorities say that the child should show signs of problems with eating, sleeping, and activity before they will diagnose depression and prescribe an antidepressant. I do not think all these symptoms necessarily need to be present for a child to be depressed.

**TREATING CHILDREN WITH DEPRESSION**   It is preferable to try to treat childhood depression with psychotherapy, which should include the whole family, before trying medication. Children have much more plasticity; it is easier to help them change attitudes and behaviors than it is with adults. Childhood depressions may respond to treatment in a relatively short amount of time. (See Chapter 13 for a description of various kinds of psychotherapy.)

I find that some depressed children can be successfully treated with antidepressants, even though I know that they would do even better if their parents could afford psychotherapy. (Many children need antidepressants even though they are in psychotherapy because the psychotherapy is not working well enough.)

The antidepressants I have prescribed and work well to relieve childhood depression are imipramine (Tofranil), nortriptyline (Pamelor), and desipramine (Norpramin). They are safe if used appropriately. If your doctor also prescribes them, ask him if he is going to test blood levels to see if they are too low, too high, or therapeutic. You should also ask him to obtain electrocardiograms during treatment as a precaution against complications.

## ANXIETY DISORDERS OF CHILDHOOD AND ADOLESCENCE

During childhood and adolescence three types of anxiety can prove troublesome to the point of being considered disorders: the inability of a child to tolerate separation from a parent, the related problem with children who shrink from others and withdraw into the family, and the child who is overanxious.

Other syndromes that are often confused with anxiety disorders in childhood and adolescence include:

*Attention deficit disorder with hyperactivity.* An anxious child will be able to concentrate in a safe setting. The hyperactive child's behavior is rarely affected by how secure he feels. (This will be discussed in greater detail below.)

*Conduct disorder.* Both an anxious child and a child with conduct disorder may both be truant from school. Usually the anxious child will stay at home because of separation anxiety, while the child with conduct disorder will stay away from home because he is not particularly anxious about separation.

*Cocaine and amphetamine abuse.* These drugs can make children anxious, and we are seeing their abuse in younger and younger children—even in seven- and eight-year-olds.

*Tourette's disorder.* If a child has mild tics without vocalizations, he may be labeled "nervous." However, most antianxiety treatments will not have an effect on this problem.

*Hyperthyroidism*
*Irritable Bowel Syndrome*

Diagnosing anxiety disorder in children is time-consuming and expensive, since your doctor has to carefully rule out organic causes before diagnosing your child's problem as anxiety. In this era of cost containment, insurance companies are often reluctant to pay for the testing necessary to arrive at a psychological diagnosis. And physicians, because of their training, may tend to treat the physical symptoms (upset stomach, headache) rather than the underlying psychological cause.

**SEPARATION ANXIETY**　Many children are afraid to leave their parents, particularly when they first go off to school or preschool. Usually this anxiety passes very quickly. When it is intense, the child may scream and cannot bear to be left, especially by the mother. If this happens repeatedly, the child may have a separation anxiety disorder. Besides being afraid to go to school, the child may be overly clinging and dependent, afraid to sleep alone, and excessively preoccupied with real or fantasized dangers to the integrity of the family unit.

He may worry about being lost and never reunited with his family. He may be afraid of the dark and worry about monsters attacking at an age when these fears are not appropriate.

As with many other disorders, children can have a weak or strong predisposition to develop separation anxiety. That is why some children develop it no matter what and others require a severe life stress, such as loss of a loved one or a pet, for it to occur.

Many people seem to think that this disorder occurs because of broken homes, but that does not appear to be the case. I have long felt that there is a biologic tendency to develop anxiety on separation because it occurs more often in the close-knit family than in the neglected child. The actual reason for the disorder may be dysfunction of a part of the limbic system of the brain.

**Treating Separation Anxiety**　There are several ways to treat separation anxiety; psychological treatment emphasizing family therapy is undoubtedly the best. If it is unavailable, however, the disorder can be treated with drugs. The medication most often prescribed has traditionally been the antidepressant imipramine (Tofranil), which usually works fairly well.

**AVOIDANCE ANXIETY**　This type of anxiety involves an excessive shrinking from contact with unfamiliar people and a desire for relationships only with family members and peers the child or adolescent knows well.

Certainly this behavior occurs in all children at one time or another. But some children are overanxious as well. If the problem is severe, the child may have an avoidant personality disorder. These children are usually timid and feel very uncomfortable in social situations. They have few friends and are considered wallflowers.

This problem is generated from within, rarely from without. It has very little to do with a child's appearance or physical abilities or even with how dysfunctional the family is. Although in traditional middle-class settings athletic ability in boys and physical attractiveness in girls are thought to be two of the more obvious keys to social success, in truth much of such success is actually determined by the personality of the child. The good news is that the characteristics of a child's personality are not immutable and may be modified, particularly when the child is suffering from avoidant disorder. The bad news is that many behaviors appear to be genetically predetermined and have little to do with environmental influences. Studies of twins separated at birth reveal startling behavioral similarities between them as adults.

**Treating Avoidance Anxiety**   Today's tendency to refer problems such as avoidance anxiety to psychologists is actually beneficial in these cases, since behavioral therapy is often very effective. The trouble is that the doctors who do the referring often ignore the fact that a great many families do not have the financial means to afford such treatments. If your insurance doesn't cover psychotherapy, ask the counselor at your child's school for a referral to a low-cost community health clinic. Many accept reduced fees.

If no psychotherapy is available, the alternative treatment by drugs is effective and comparatively inexpensive, although drugs don't help resolve life or family situations that may be triggering the anxiety. Medications are often strikingly effective by themselves and should be considered if your doctor suggests psychotherapy you cannot afford.

Find a doctor who understands pharmacology well and who will work with you. Your doctor must be very careful about what drugs he uses in children. I do not use anxiety-reducing drugs called benzodiazepines in children (Valium, Xanax, Ativan, etc.) except in very special situations because they are addictive.

Other medications that increase brain serotonin (a chemical involved in nerve transmissions), such as some of the antidepressants, seem to be very effective.

I have also found that a monoamine oxidase inhibitor (MAOI) which acts to ease both anxiety as well as depression, works well for avoidance anxiety, although your doctor may want to use the drug fluoxetine (Prozac) first, since it has fewer potential adverse reactions. (The adverse reactions of Prozac include nervousness, insomnia, and intestinal distress. If a rash occurs, the drug should be stopped immediately. Prozac can occasionally make depression worse, and also cause patients to become angry or hostile.) Even though MAOIs are safe if used properly, I will only prescribe them for teenagers who appear to be responsible people, since serious adverse reactions can occur if certain rules about foods and other medications are not followed.

Where anxiety in children is concerned, I believe in intervening as early as possible, not only to eliminate unnecessary misery and suffering but also so that the important years of personality development in school will not be impaired as well. Be wary of doctors who lightly dismiss the problem with "He'll outgrow it." The saddest part of such an unwarranted dismissal of a child's problem is that it can be so readily treated.

**OVERANXIOUSNESS**   Overanxious children worry about almost everything. It is natural for a child to worry when it's time for an exam or when some stressful situation is coming up—the first day of school or going to the doctor's office. However, when the anxiety is extreme and repeated, the problem may be overanxious disorder. These children are always tense and self-conscious. They appear sad and are worried about anything and everything you can imagine. They need professional help.

Sometimes these children are diagnosed as having another problem, attention deficit disorder (which we'll be discussing next), because they do not concentrate well. As a result they are given stimulants. However, children with overanxious disorder will become even more anxious if they are given stimulants. It's important to know that overanxious disorder is quite common in children and is also underdiagnosed.

If your child is a worrier about everything and your doctor concludes he actually has attention deficit disorder and prescribes a stimulant, be sure to ask about anxiety. If the stimulant makes him even more anxious, you should go back to your doctor immediately and discuss alternative diagnoses.

**Treating Overanxious Disorder**   I tend to treat these children the same way I do adults with generalized anxiety disorder, with antidepressants (except that I do not use benzodiazepines). Also, schools often have counselors who are skilled in group therapy, where children can discuss their anxieties and fears and learn to cope with them.

## HYPERACTIVITY

Many people, especially parents, use the word *hyperactivity* without really understanding the behavior they are trying to describe. *Hyperactivity* has become a kind of generic term for whenever Johnny doesn't do well in school. A typical description is that he is a poor learner.

In some cases the problem is short-lived and could be caused by problems at home or by a variety of other illnesses. Usually these incidental hyperactive states can be treated by most doctors who take the time to search for the underlying cause. Family systems therapy with some behavior modification may resolve the problem if it is not primarily organic.

On the other hand, if the symptoms continue and Johnny is constantly restless, unable to pay attention, and makes it difficult for those around to concentrate on their work, a physical cause should be considered.

This sort of hyperactivity is thought to be caused by a part of the brain that is not working properly. This disorder, which occurs most commonly in children, can make Johnny's life miserable and keep him from developing friends or excelling intellectually. It can also drive his parents to distraction. (Hyperactivity is technically Attention Deficit/Hyperactivity Disorder, or ADHD. Attention deficit disorder has two variations, one with hyperactivity, the other without. Some 3 to 5 percent of children in the United States are estimated to have this illness.)

The good news is that, correctly diagnosed, ADHD is treatable. The bad news is that it is sometimes linked in children and a few adults with the associated problem, conduct disorder.

**MISDIAGNOSIS**	The parent of an ADHD child faces the problem of correct diagnosis. The condition can be confused with several other physical and emotional disorders, all of which a good physician must eliminate before diagnosing ADHD.

Watch out for a quick diagnosis in schools made by undertrained and overworked counselors. It may turn out that your child does not have ADHD or an associated medical problem but may instead be suffering from a learning disorder such as dyslexia, which prevents him from understanding what he reads. (To complicate matters, many patients with ADHD also have a learning disorder.) Or he may be overanxious, reflecting family stresses at home.

A tip-off to a misdiagnosis of ADHD is the child who is hyperactive at home but not in school. A dysfunctional family can produce in a child hyperactive behavior that normalizes in a structured classroom setting. This form of emotionally hyperactive behavior cannot be distinguished from any other type.

Schools sometimes want the doctor to put the child on a drug like methylphenidate (Ritalin) to control his behavior, so that he will be less of a classroom disruption and can learn more easily. There is no convincing evidence that he (many more boys than girls have ADHD) will learn more when on this drug, but some doctors simply take the easy way out and do what the school or parents want.

I see many adults with attention deficit disorder which was never diagnosed, and more than one patient has broken down crying in my office after successful treatment when he realized how his life had been wasted because of that lack of diagnosis. Often they are intelligent people who have only been able to work at low-level occupations because of their problem. Now, late in life, it may be very difficult or impossible, because of family responsibilities or other life situations, to do much about it.

Many children or adults with attention deficit/hyperactivity disorder may also develop impulse control disorders later in life. They are prone to develop compulsions involving gambling, kleptomania, and sexual acting-out.

A person with this problem often has adult relatives with the same disorder. The family members also may have antisocial personalities and other psychiatric disorders. Often the parents are divorced; sometimes the father is in jail or engaged in illegal activities. The single mother who is not affected may be overwhelmed with her responsibilities and problems.

**ILLNESSES OFTEN CONFUSED WITH ADHD** Attention deficit disorder with or without hyperactivity is often misdiagnosed because of a chaotic family environment, although most of my patients with this problem are children of solid citizens who are bewildered and frustrated by the situation. A chaotic family environment can produce inattention, hyperactive behavior, and impulsivity by itself. In addition, here are some conditions with which this disorder is most often confused:

Anxiety
Depression
Mania
Pervasive developmental disorder
Seizure disorders
Overactive thyroid
Pinworms
Learning disorder
Vision or hearing impairment
Tourette's disorder
Food or environmental allergies
Child abuse
Mental retardation
Lead poisoning

**DIAGNOSIS** If you suspect your child may have attention deficit/hyperactivity disorder, you will want a thorough diagnosis. The main diagnostic scale used by teachers and is usually handed to me by a parent who brings her child in for treatment is the Conners 39-item scale, a way of rating classroom behavior. Unfortunately, nobody I know and nothing

I've read in the literature I have reviewed likes it very much. Its results are questionable.

There are other tests, but they are longer and harder to administer. To get a really good diagnosis, a sophisticated assessment battery must be given, but many school psychologists are minimally trained to perform these tests, even if they had time to do them. (Many schools are so underfunded that only children with the most severe disorders get this kind of evaluation.)

**BEHAVIORS CHARACTERISTIC OF ADHD**   The most common ADHD behaviors, according to *DSM-III-R*, are being fidgety, not sitting still, being easily distracted, having difficulty waiting a turn in games or group situations, blurting out answers, not finishing tasks, and talking loudly and excessively. The core behaviors are inability to sustain attention, hyperactivity, and impulsiveness.

Other diagnoses your doctor should particularly consider are pervasive developmental disorder (PDD), in which a child does not relate well to others and has impaired communication skills. Severe ADHD may overlap with PDD; the two disorders are not distinct in some situations.

Those with PDD (a severe impairment that includes infantile autism) may behave in a stereotyped (repetitive) manner, do not engage in interpersonal behaviors, and have distinctive rigidities in conversational speech.

Tourette's disorder can coexist with ADHD or occur separately. The diagnosis would be important for your doctor to establish, since the treatment of ADHD can make the tics of Tourette's disorder worse if stimulants are used.

**ADD WITH HYPERACTIVITY**   It is not hard for me to diagnose the attention deficit disorder *with* hyperactivity in a child who is bouncing off my office walls, picking things up and putting them down, and jumping from one topic to another during conversation. But many of these children appear fairly normal in a one-to-one situation and can even watch a Saturday morning cartoon show all the way through—well, almost.

**ADD WITHOUT HYPERACTIVITY**   The child with attention deficit disorder *without* hyperactivity is harder to diagnose at first and may be thought to be just "slow" or daydreaming since he does not fight with his peers or disrupt the class.

Since it is so important to make an accurate diagnosis, it puzzles me that hardly anyone knows how easy it is to do with a procedure called a BEAM scan. A BEAM scan is a form of topographic brain mapping in which EEG (brain-wave) data and "evoked responses" (reactions to a stimulus to the eye, ear, or body) are electrically followed through the brain, analyzed by a computer, and displayed on an image of the head seen from above.

People with pure attention deficit disorder will lack or have an abnormality in one kind of evoked response that is present in "normal" people. BEAM scans are helpful because they distinguish ADD or ADHD from similar illnesses. Scans that measure brain blood flow can also be helpful in making the diagnosis: in ADHD one region of the brain may be abnormal.

**TREATING THE PROBLEM**  No one knows why either children or adults get this disorder, although there is a slight hereditary tendency toward it. However, the disorder disappears on its own during adolescence in about half the children who have it.

Behavioral therapy is best done on a situation-by-situation basis. The most difficult situation for children with this disorder is in the classroom, where they are asked to sit still and concentrate—something they simply cannot do. Many teachers simply do not know what to do with these children, and physicians often do not have the time to provide direction.

Here are some recommendations that may help a teacher cope with a child with ADHD:

1. Keep directions short.
2. Do not give more than one direction at a time.
3. Ask the child to repeat the directions.
4. Keep distractions to a minimum during study time by using a carrel (a three-sided box that fits on the child's desk so that he cannot be disturbed by his neighbors).
5. Provide frequent breaks.
6. If possible, let the child exercise during the breaks (run an errand to the office, etc.).
7. Try to determine which learning channel is most efficient

for the child and emphasize that channel to reduce frustration. Usually a child has a preferred channel, whether audio, visual, or kinesthetic.

8. If the child also seems to have a learning disorder, refer him to the school reading specialist or school psychologist for evaluation.

9. Provide prompt feedback for written work to a child with ADHD. Giving back a corrected paper two or three days later is nearly meaningless to these children.

10. Keep tasks short. The ADHD child cannot sit for long periods of time without his attention wandering.

11. The ADHD child gets a lot of negative feedback regarding behavior. Although it is hard to ignore negative behavior and some negative behavior just can't be ignored, provide positive feedback when possible.

12. When the child begins to act out, provide "time out." Have the child go for a short period of time to a desk at the back of the room where distractions are minimal and he can get his act together.

13. Remember, an ADHD child has few internal controls. Provide more structure for him, such as a set schedule each day.

14. Establish a system of rewards for appropriate behavior.

15. Remember that the child with ADHD is usually unintentionally overactive and distractible. Often he is dismayed by his own behavior and needs to be reassured that he is cared for in spite of his behavior problems.

16. Enlist the help of teacher aides and school counselors to provide guidance and support.

17. Communicate clearly with the child's family. Usually they are as concerned as you are, particularly when the child also does poorly in school academics. (If the child appears to have a poor home support system, the child needs you to be stable and caring more than ever.) Send short notes home when the child has had success or a good day, not only when discipline is needed.

Recommendations that may help parents cope with a child with ADHD include:

1. Follow many of the directions listed above. Keep family life as organized and calm as possible. Remember the ADHD child has few internal controls and needs structure and scheduling more than most children.
2. If the child reads, write lists of tasks for him to do each day (empty the trash, clean his room, etc.). Making a chart with Sunday through Saturday across the top, with tasks listed vertically along one side, will remind him to do certain chores on certain days. Put an X on the day you wish the task done.
3. Set up a reward system. Try to avoid a reward system based on objects as much as possible. Other rewards include short trips (zoo, park, etc.) or seeing a movie. Reward task completion and length of time spent in active concentration on a task.
4. Be watchful for sibling jealousy. Siblings may perceive that their brother or sister is getting preferential treatment. Often a family will shower attention on a child with special needs and unintentionally neglect a sibling. As hard as it can be, try not to take a well-balanced achieving sibling for granted.
5. Keep oral directions short and speak slowly.
6. Keep home distractions minimal by limiting the number of playmates he can have over at one time and encouraging him to engage in quiet activities.
7. As hard as it is to avoid the use of negatives, try to reward positive behavior and ignore negative behavior. Eventually, an ADHD child will see any attention as a reinforcer, so concentrate on rewarding positive behavior.
8. Build your child's self-esteem. Encourage him to set behavioral and academic goals that he can meet.
9. Provide organized outlets for his excess energy. Try to channel it in a positive direction through sports or group activities emphasizing service to others.
10. Avail yourself of help from local or national support groups for parents of learning-disabled children. They are excellent sources of advice and will help you deal effectively with school-based problems.

11. Help the child understand that it is his behavior that is the
    problem, that he is loved apart from his behavior.

It's important to understand that the child's excess activity
cannot be eliminated, but it can be kept under control with the
above and similar measures.

The parents who follow these suggestions may be rewarded
by much-improved behavior. They may, in fact, believe that
they are "out of the woods." Sending their child to camp for
a week or a visit to Granny, however, will quickly remove that
delusion. In a week or two all their accomplishments may be
undone.

**FOOD THERAPY**   Most parents prefer to go with the least
radical therapy first. This may involve various restriction diets
or megavitamin therapy before using drugs. Unfortunately,
these methods tend to be difficult to comply with, are time-
consuming, and seldom work.

**MULTIMODAL TREATMENT**   It is better if the treatment
is multimodal: many different methods of teaching the child
are attempted both at home by parents and at school by teachers. Medication may be prescribed by your doctor as well as
using ways described in the lists above to reduce distraction
and enhance learning.

Medication used alone, however, can be quite effective.
Medication helps about 75 percent of the children, although
how it works is still poorly understood.

**TREATMENT WITH MEDICINE**   It may be difficult to
think of giving drugs to children. There is, of course, enormous
and justifiable concern over drug abuse. There is also considerable publicity suggesting that many medications are overprescribed. Is it any wonder that many parents say "I don't
want my child taking drugs!"?

However, allowing your doctor to give a medication that
corrects an unwanted behavior is not the same as giving heroin
or cocaine. And if drugs are all your doctor has left in his
arsenal, you may not have a choice. In reality, drugs aren't so
bad, considering the alternative of having an unhappy child

with poor peer relations and low self-esteem, practically a blueprint for future problems.

I often try a harmless sugar pill (a placebo) first to see if simply taking any medication will do the trick. If it doesn't, then there are always the active drugs to consider.

I usually start a patient with ADHD on a prescription antidepressant called desipramine (Norpramin). It often works very well in doses considerably lower than those used for depression. It has the added benefit that if your child is depressed, it will also help. If your doctor misses the diagnosis (because of subtlety, time, money, and because BEAM scans have not yet been well standardized for those younger than nine) and instead calls the problem depression, the drug may still work, although in treating depression the physician may raise the dose to therapeutic antidepressant levels.

Norpramin is a safe drug, tolerance does not develop to it, it can be prescribed for decades, and it does not require a special triplicate prescription form (which intimidates doctors). It is also usually taken only once a day unless high doses are required, which makes it easier to get your child to take it.

There has been some recent alarm about using Norpramin in children; three sudden deaths have been reported since 1987. I consider these flukes, since imipramine (Tofranil) has been extensively used in children for many years. Its main metabolic product is desipramine.

When prescribing these antidepressants for children, I check blood levels of the medication to make sure that the dose is not too high. I also do an electrocardiogram after beginning treatment, since if these deaths were caused by Norpramin, probably the heartbeat was irregular or too fast. If the electrocardiogram is abnormal, I may stop the drug and repeat it in a few weeks to see if the abnormality was resolved. (Parents may beg me not to stop the medication, but under these circumstances it would be prudent to do so.) You will want to ask your physician if he is likewise taking these precautions. Any drug use must be closely monitored by your physician.

Methylphenidate (Ritalin) can also be effective. However, your doctor may hesitate to prescribe it because it needs to be given three or four times a day and can cause insomnia if given after 6:00 P.M. There is a sustained-release form of Ritalin, but some experts think it does not work quite as well. Ritalin is the most frequently prescribed medication for ADHD; however, many physicians and psychologists believe it is overprescribed. Side effects may include insomnia, decreased appetite, and (according to some) slightly shorter stature if taken for many years.

Dextroamphetamine (Dexedrine) can be given less frequently than Ritalin (it may be given only once or twice a day) and works as well. It is not favored over Ritalin, however, because it has more side effects.

Your doctor may be hesitant to prescribe either Ritalin or Dexedrine because of the possibility they could be abused either by your child or by friends or relatives to whom he might give the drug. If your doctor feels that they are the drugs of choice, you should assure him that you and your child will not abuse the substance.

Pemoline (Cylert) is a stimulant that also may be helpful. It is not a controlled substance, but it takes two or three weeks to work. It can be harmful to the liver, so periodic blood tests are recommended. (Cylert causes liver problems more often in adults than in children, but not very often in either.)

**SIDE EFFECTS**   The medications discussed are called stimulants and *all* stimulants can cause tics—minor spasms or jerky movements of various parts of the body. There has been a worry that they can induce a certain kind of severe tic disorder called Tourette's disorder (see Chapter 11), but that concern usually is not justified. The tics almost always resolve when the stimulants are stopped. Nevertheless, many doctors will not prescribe stimulants if there is a family history of Tourette's disorder or if they think your child might already have a minor tic disorder.

**OTHER MEDICATIONS**   The stimulants noted above all have different pharmacologic modes of action and all should probably be tried in difficult cases. In addition, there is another class of stimulants that are quite safe and do not require triplicate prescriptions. They are unfortunately often totally ignored by physicians.

If your doctor is hesitant to prescribe the medications noted above, you may want to suggest these. They fall under the general heading of diet pills or appetite suppressants. I like phentermine (Ionamin). Ionamin does not give most people a buzz, is not generally abused, and whatever appetite suppression it causes usually lasts only a few weeks.

DDAVP (des-amino d-arginine vasopressin) is a safe compound that is sprayed into the nose once or twice a day. The only possible side effects are headache, nausea, and occasional water retention, and the dosage can be reduced or the drug stopped if adverse reactions occur. I described its use years ago in ADHD and my work has been confirmed by others. It does not cause tics and is not abused. I do not know why it is not used more often, but you cannot even find its use described in most review articles on the illness.

**WHEN STIMULANTS DON'T WORK**   Some children get worse on stimulants. This response can be a problem if your doctor doesn't understand it and instead prescribes increasingly higher dosages of the stimulants.

If the stimulants don't work, you can suggest that your doctor try the opposite tack. I use a drug that acts in an opposite way. It's called verapamil (Calan, Isoptin) and is a calcium channel blocker. Verapamil is the most frequently prescribed calcium channel blocker for children, usually given for heart problems but sometimes effective in stimulant-resistant ADHD. Drugs called monoamine oxidase inhibitors (MAOIs) have also been found effective and are sometimes prescribed. I hesitate giving them to children with ADHD since certain foods and medications can cause serious adverse reactions in a patient who is taking an MAOI. And since children and teenagers are noncompliant by nature—hyperactive patients particularly so—prescribing an MAOI for them is a risk.

Some promising treatments your doctor may want to consider, if all else fails, include: buspirone (Buspar), an antianxiety medication with other potential uses, especially in impulse-control disorders; and buproprion (Wellbutrin), an antidepressant, which may be effective but should not be given to children. If you take your Wellbutrin doses too close together there is a small possibility of having a seizure. It should be used with great caution in those with seizure disorders or a history of serious head injuries.

## BEDWETTING

Wetting the bed during the night (enuresis) is something all children do until control of the urinary bladder is achieved—for most children by three or four years of age. In some children (about 10 percent), however, control is not attained until much later, with much resultant distress to both child and parents.

Fortunately, the older the child, the more likely bedwetting will stop on its own. In short, if you can stand it and don't blame the child for it, most bedwetting will eventually go away.

Unfortunately, this degree of tolerance is not found in many families, and therefore two difficulties may arise. The first is that, even though the doctor may not find a problem, if you are concerned, your worry makes the bedwetting a problem that must be dealt with. If nothing is done, your child's self-image may suffer.

The other problem is that your physician may immediately resort to drug therapy, although if everyone simply waited a while, perhaps as short a time as a few months, the whole problem might disappear.

How do you know what is appropriate treatment?

First, if you are concerned that something serious is wrong, ask the doctor to do a work-up. Tests can be taken to establish that there aren't any underlying physical problems (like a urinary infection) that are resulting the bedwetting. Disorders your doctor will investigate are:

Kidney disease or infection
Bladder disease or infection
Malformations of the urinary tract

If your child had any of the above disorders, however, he or she would probably wet during the day as well as the night. If your child wets only during the night, most likely the problem is not any of these.

Once urinary-tract disorders have been ruled out, you can

do some simple things to help your child overcome the problem. The first thing you can do is understand what causes bedwetting.

**WHAT CAUSES BEDWETTING?**   A common theory has been that bedwetting is the result of some sort of a maturational lag in the control of the brain over bladder emptying. This is a fairly reasonable idea, but one that has been difficult to prove.

Bedwetting has also been divided into the kind that has persisted since infancy (primary) and the type that recurs after the child has been dry at night for at least six months (secondary). Secondary bedwetting is likely to be due to diseases or, much more commonly, emotional problems in the child such as regression when a new baby brother or sister arrives or upon moving to a new house.

Primary bedwetting, the kind that has persisted since infancy, can be due to the child's having a smaller functional bladder capacity than is normal for his or her age. When the bladder fills to a certain point it begins to contract so that it will empty. The bladders of bedwetting children probably begin to contract sooner than they should. The result is involuntary wetting. These children's bladders tend not to tighten the external sphincter (the muscle that voluntarily controls the release of urine) while asleep.

Most children and adults wake up when they have to urinate. Bedwetting children apparently respond to these signals less readily. They may also have a disturbed secretion of a brain hormone, vasopressin, which regulates the production of more urine.

**The Importance of Treatment**   Unfortunately, in some cases bedwetting that does not clear up at an appropriate age can have a severe effect on children's lives. I have treated several young men and women in their late teens and early twenties who had primary enuresis that had been a shameful "family secret." Trying to hide the disorder had resulted in a significant alteration of their lives and levels of self-esteem. It is a shame, since the situation does not have to occur; treatment is fairly straightforward and almost always successful, at least in my experience.

**TREATING BEDWETTING**   Once you understand that the problem is probably one of maturity (primary) or emotion (secondary), you can take action. Secondary bedwetters may require some behavioral or supportive therapy. Primary bedwetters (those who have never stopped), however, usually receive little benefit from psychotherapy except for coping with feelings of shame.

Your family doctor or pediatrician, if well informed and if he or she has the time or personnel to do it, can instruct you on techniques of training your child to increase bladder volume without urinating and increasing the strength of the external sphincter muscle of the urethra (the tube leading out of the bladder).

On your own, for a nominal amount you can purchase one of several alarms that sound when wetting occurs. These condition the child to wake up upon urinating. If used in a positive way ("This device will help you do what you want to do") and without any negative feedback added ("This is punishment for your bad action"), they can be quite effective.

In addition, the child can also be motivated in various ways to stop bedwetting. One possibly successful technique has been hypnosis. I have never tried to hypnotize a child myself to stop bedwetting but would do so in a difficult situation. Children are usually good hypnotic subjects.

**COMBINATION OF TECHNIQUES**   Bedwetting can often be successfully managed by a combination of the described techniques as well as by making your child responsible for being dry. This is usually accomplished by *having him help wash and dry the sheets when he has wet them*. It's important, however, that this be done *not* as a punishment but to help promote a feeling of maturity and responsibility.

**MEDICATIONS**   As a last resort, your doctor may want to use various medications to treat bedwetting. These include the antidepressant imipramine (Tofranil) and oxybutynin chloride (Ditropan). No one knows exactly how Tofranil works, but Ditropan blocks the chemical that causes bladder contractions. Another that I and a number of other physicians have been using for a while is DDAVP, a synthetic variation of vasopressin, a hormone that comes from the pituitary gland in the brain and decreases the quantity of urine produced by the kidneys. All of these medications can—though rarely—have adverse reactions or may not be effective.

The important thing to remember is that children are very sensitive to criticism from a respected adult such as a parent, and this respected adult must help the child understand that while bedwetting can be annoying for all concerned, it is not shameful or a reflection on the child's character.

# Afterword

There are encouraging and discouraging trends in the future of American medicine. The status of family practice and general internal medicine is secure, but the scope of these specialties is so wide, they are intimidating. They also require longer hours for physicians than higher paying fields, and it is difficult for physicians to spend an hour or so dealing with a patient's complex problem if office overhead must be paid. General physicians must see a large number of patients in a day in order to be able to pay their bills. The alternative is to do "procedures" such as surgery or look into various orifices of the body with specialized instruments. Procedures may pay a physician ten or twenty times as much as he could earn from talking with you or examining you for the same period of time.

If medicine turns more to a form of care called "capitation," doctors will be paid a certain amount of money each month for your health care whether you are well or sick. This form of health care rewards the physician for doing as little as possible, although ideally the physician who can solve problems the most creatively and efficiently should do well in this system. If national health insurance becomes a reality, medical care will be assured for everyone. Whether this care will be so limited that it will provide mediocre medicine for all remains to be seen.

Innovative medical care will be harder to find. There will be "flow charts," recipes of how to handle every medical problem, in the next few years, much like the "cookbook" I have discussed. Medical interventions in this system which do not adhere to what has been proven by several double-blind experiments will be discouraged, perhaps protecting patients from the incompetent and the negligent, but also perhaps depriving them of creative approaches, unless they are able to pay for them privately. In some countries (Canada is a good example), patients are not allowed to pay for health care outside of the national health program, therefore many wealthier Canadians come to the United States for "special" treatment.

Nevertheless, potential health benefits have never been better. The understanding we now have of health and disease at the level of the cell and the molecule is astonishing, undreamt of when I was a medical student. Health care technology in the United States is still the envy of the rest of the world, although how long this situation will last remains to be seen because medicine is so closely tied to the state of the economy. Health care rationing is the standard of the day, and funds available for research are continually shrinking. If no money is available to do experiments to validate innovative approaches, new treatments may never reach the mainstream. Many physicians will not use any approach that is not well validated; others are afraid to do so because of potential sanctions from insurers or regulatory agencies, or because of potential malpractice suits.

We live in an era of great promise and great obstacles in medicine. I hope that this book has helped you to deal with some of the possible dilemmas you may encounter. As medicine evolves, new problems in diagnosis and treatment will continue to arise. Perhaps I shall be able to help you deal with those in a future book.

# Index